The
W.O.W.
DIET

Also by Michelle Snow
Available from Cedar Fort

It's in the Bag: A New, Easy, Affordable, and Doable Approach to Food Storage

The
W.O.W.
DIET

**WORDS OF WISDOM AND DIETARY ENLIGHTENMENT
FROM LEADING WORLD RELIGIONS AND SCIENTIFIC STUDY**

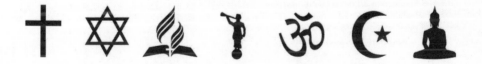

MICHELLE SNOW
RN, MSPH, MSHR, PHD (C)

BONNEVILLE BOOKS
SPRINGVILLE, UTAH

ISBN 13:978-1-59955-386-3
Published by Bonneville Books, an imprint of Cedar Fort, Inc., 2373 W. 700 S., Springville, UT 84663
Distributed by Cedar Fort, Inc., www.cedarfort.com

LIBRARY OF CONGRESS CATALOGING-IN-PUBLICATION DATA

Snow, Michelle, 1961-
  The W.O.W. Diet : words of wisdom from leading world religions / Michelle Snow.
    p. cm.
  Summary: Recipes and food suggestions for a healthy diet.
  Includes index.
  ISBN 978-1-59955-386-3
  1. Nutrition—Religious aspects. 2. Diet. I. Title.

  TX357.S58 2010
  613.2—dc22

                    2010024851

Cover design by Angela D. Olsen
Cover design © 2010 by Lyle Mortimer
Edited and typeset by Megan E. Welton

Printed in the United States of America

10 9 8 7 6 5 4 3 2 1

Printed on acid-free paper

DEDICATION

This book is lovingly dedicated to my husband, Trent.

CONTENTS

ACKNOWLEDGMENTS

I would like to thank our daughter, Rachel Snow, and the skilled employees of Cedar Fort Publishing for their assistance in publishing this book.

PREFACE:

WHAT DO YOU WANT OUT OF FOOD?

I f I were to ask you what characteristics ideal foods possess, I would expect the following responses:

- TASTE—The food must taste delicious.
- NUTRITION—The food must have vitamins and nutrients beneficial for good health.
- NON FATTENING—The food needs to help me maintain or lose weight without leaving me hungry!
- VALUE—The food shouldn't break the bank.
- CONVENIENCE—The food must be quick and easy to prepare.

What if I told you that I discovered foods that meet all of the above criteria and that they have been in existence for millennia? Join me as I share with you my personal journey toward dietary enlightenment—a journey which resulted in an alleviation of my gastrointestinal problems, significant and sustained weight loss, lower cholesterol, and increased vitality.

When I first started researching religious dietary doctrines in 2006, I searched the Internet for authorized websites of religious organizations that I knew followed dietary laws. I also searched scholarly publications using keywords as well as the local and university libraries. I had no idea that I would write a book detailing my journey, so I only wrote down the information that I found pertinent and did not save the references. Having said this, the following summary consists of major religions and their dietary guidelines. Please note that this information is not intended to be all-encompassing; however, the references used are readily available on the Internet and were accessed in 2009–2010. I have included references to the books I've read to gain further understanding of the religions and the accompanying dietary observances. You will find these references in a comprehensive bibliography at the end of this book.

CHAPTER ONE:

REGULARLY
IRREGULAR

In 1976, I was sitting at the kitchen bar, eating a snack, when I overheard a conversation between my mother and her friend Marie.

"Dianne," Marie said. "Bridgette only has a bowel movement once a week. Do you think I should take her to the doctor?"

"Really?" my mother, Dianne, responded in an anxious voice. "You better call the doctor and get her in as fast as you can. At her age, she might have a blockage or something. This happens with older people." Bridgette was Marie's eighty-something-year-old mother-in-law who happened to be visiting from Belgium.

It wasn't until that moment that I realized having a bowel movement just once or twice a month wasn't normal. Once Marie left, I approached my mother and quizzed her about regularity. After answering a few questions, she asked why I was concerned about defecation. I told her that I had overheard her conversation with Marie and that I didn't even have a bowel movement once a week. She told me to increase my fruit and vegetable intake, exercise, and drink lots of water, and all would be fine.

I was an athletic girl who swam in our pool nearly every day in the summer, skied in the winter, played baseball in the city league, and enjoyed racquetball and basketball a couple times a week with my dad and brother. I followed my mom's advice and began drinking more water and eating extra helpings of fruit and vegetables. I even took up jogging. And as you have probably already guessed—because this book is more than a few pages in length—nothing changed, and I never brought the embarrassing subject up again.

After graduating from high school, I initially decided on a career as a registered nurse, which provided the means for me to pursue my terminal degree of a PhD in public health. My constipation problems continued throughout college. Years ago, I visited my family practitioner and discussed my constipation with him. He, like my mother, confidently said, "Increase your exercise, fiber, and water intake." And then he disparagingly added as he stood by the door, "Michelle, with your background, you of all people should know how to treat constipation." He was right—being a nurse and having degrees in public health meant that I *did* know about diet, exercise, bowel training, and laxatives. I was also keenly aware of the diseases and conditions that might develop as a result of prolonged constipation.

In an effort to have a bowel movement, I tried many things. I placed myself on a bowel-training program. I used a wide variety of fiber supplements and still nothing happened. I went vegan on three separate occasions for about six months each time. If I saw a cow after five months on a vegan diet, I would respond much like Alex the lion on the movie *Madagascar* when his zebra pal, Marty, transforms into a steak. I nearly had to stop myself from running out in the field and chewing on the poor cow's hind quarters. After three failed attempts at veganism, I decided to never attempt a vegan diet again. Still, I jogged and even tried imagery, but my bowel habits worsened.

I could not defecate without taking extreme measures. Most people will have a bowel movement if they take two laxative tablets—I was taking up to *six* tablets with minimal results. Eventually, I turned to magnesium citrate, which is a strong oral laxative that is commonly used to cleanse the intestines before bowel surgery or a colonoscopy. Magnesium citrate worked but not without side effects: I would be confined to the bathroom for at least a full day.

In my forties, my abdomen was distended to the point that I looked five months pregnant. My stomach hurt incessantly. I felt like I was going to vomit at any moment. I was hungry but felt even worse after meals, and I frequently belched but rarely passed flatulence. One night, I could no longer handle the abdominal pain in my lower right quadrant. I thought I was developing appendicitis. I was admitted to the emergency department, but the physician ruled out appendicitis. He said that there was definitely something wrong, but he didn't know what it was. He further instructed me to return to the emergency department if my condition worsened or if I developed a fever. I didn't develop a fever, so I never went back.

Years later, I met a young woman who was recovering from a colonostomy. She could not say enough good things about her gastroenterologist. I eagerly made an appointment and was scheduled for a colonoscopy. Unfortunately, after the colonoscopy was performed, the gastroenterologist found no blockage, growths, tumors, or polyps, but he did offer me two prescriptions to increase bowel motility. As I was leaving the office, he casually added that I may have celiac disease or irritable bowel syndrome (IBS). He said that I should try a gluten-free diet for a month. If my symptoms abated, I had celiac disease. He added that if I didn't get relief from a gluten-free diet, I should try eliminating any foods that exacerbated my symptoms, as there was no specific diet for IBS. I left the medical building discouraged and feeling as though I had exhausted all of my options.

Little did I know that being disappointed in the outcome of a doctor's appointment would lead me on a path to dietary enlightenment and health! Later, after tearfully explaining to my husband that I was once again at a dead end, he simply said. "Michelle, have you ever prayed to see what God has to say about your condition?" I've prayed to God since I was a child, but I never once asked Him about the cause of my severe constipation. I had never thought to pray to God about something as disgusting as stool or, in my case, a lack of stool.

I looked at my husband, laughed, spouted off a few bawdy remarks about being "full of it," and went about my day. As the day passed, my husband's suggestion kept running through my mind. Halfheartedly, I went to my room, entered my closet, and tried to speak to God about my long-standing constipation. To say the least, I felt awkward. In my mind, my prayer seemed improper. I prefaced my prayer by apologizing in an attempt not to offend.

I explained to God my condition and recited to Him all of my efforts to gain relief. I started crying as I explained how horrible I felt and began begging for a solution. I remember saying, "Heavenly Father, whatever I need to do, I will do it. Just tell me what it is." This was a very difficult thing for me to say because I do not like feeling vulnerable or dependent, nor am I inclined to promise to do anything without getting all of the details.

After I finished praying, I quietly lingered, and a few simple thoughts came to mind. My first thought was that I should explore celiac disease and go on a gluten-free diet for a month, and if that didn't work, I should research irritable bowel syndrome. Secondly, I had the thought to explore dietary principles shared by major religions of the world. I wondered if these principles would be scientifically supported by modern research. I am a Christian who happens to be educated and trained in science; perhaps I was being spiritually prompted to find the answers to my prayer by combining both of my worlds. I decided to find out.

I sat down at my desk and developed a research plan. The first step would be to identify religions that had dietary observances and restraints. I chose to examine Buddhism, Hinduism, Judaism, Islam, the Seventh-day Adventist Church, and the Church of Jesus Christ of Latter-day Saints (the "Mormons") for dietary guidance. I would also identify, if available, any scholarly, peer-reviewed, and published scientific studies that focused on the overall health of members from these religious groups. After analyzing the data, I would develop a doctrine-based diet and strictly adhere to it for a month to see if it would help my condition.

CHAPTER TWO:

THE SEARCH FOR
A DIAGNOSIS

All journeys have many stops: some are dead ends, some cause detours, and others lead to your desired destination. My journey to dietary health and enlightenment was no different.

STOP ONE: CELIAC DISEASE

"Celiac disease would be a nice diagnosis," I remember thinking. "All I need to do is eliminate wheat from my diet. How difficult can that be?" What ignorance! Wheat and wheat by-products are hidden in entrées, sauces, condiments, seasonings, and everything else you can think of!

Through my studies, I further learned that other grains besides wheat contain gluten. The grains or flours I could eat were amaranth, arrowroot, brown rice, buckwheat, cornmeal, maize, millet, potato, quinoa, white rice, tapioca, and teff. I could not eat rye, barley, wheat, spelt, or kamut. There appeared to be some differences of opinion among physicians regarding oats, so to be safe, I avoided oats as well. I searched the library and Internet for recipes and information about signs and symptoms of celiac disease.

As a side note, I had decided beforehand that if I did indeed have celiac disease, I would not refer to it as such—I do not particularly like the negative connotation that is associated with the word disease! Instead, I decided I would communicate my dietary restrictions to others in terms of being gluten intolerant.

I am a checklist person. If I need to make a decision, I write out the pros and cons of the different options or ways to respond to a decision. It should be no surprise that I made a gluten intolerance symptom list and proceeded to check off the symptoms I had. Remember, this list is from memory, and as such, is not all encompassing. For current gluten intolerance information, I recommend the Celiac Sprue Association website: http://www.csaceliacs.org/index.php

MY GLUTEN INTOLERANCE SYMPTOMS

Abdominal cramping	Yes
Abdominal pain	Yes
Abdominal distention	Yes
Increased appetite	No
Cravings	Sometimes hungry for some unknown something
Back pain	No
Constipation	Yes
Diarrhea	Definitely not
Flatus	No
Dry skin	No
Weight loss	No
Fatigue	No
Depression	No
Headache	1 to 3 migraines per month
Irritability	On occasion

After comparing my symptoms with the symptoms of gluten intolerance, I sincerely doubted that I was suffering from gluten intolerance. Still, I wasn't 100 percent certain because celiac disease is also named the "great imitator." It mimics the signs and symptoms of other conditions and diseases. I finally decided to commit to a gluten-free diet when I read that many people who have been diagnosed with gluten intolerance were asymptomatic. During the course of my research, I read that a biopsy of the intestine could definitively diagnose gluten intolerance.

I immediately called the gastroenterologist's office. When the nurse returned my call, she said that the doctor recommended I first try a thirty-day gluten-free diet, and if it reduced my symptoms, then he would perform a biopsy.

So, I became an avid reader of ingredient lists. I might add that reading ingredient lists takes time; this new activity increased the time I spent at the grocery store by 45 minutes or more. In an effort to save time, I searched for prepared gluten-free foods and mixes. At the time, neighborhood grocery stores didn't carry gluten-free products, and when I did find a health food store that carried something gluten-free, there wasn't much of a selection, and the cost was easily four to five times what I would normally pay for products containing gluten.

Eventually, my frugality was lost to convenience, and I broke down and purchased some gluten-free products. I vividly remember the first time I baked bread from a gluten-free mix. My family was gathered in the kitchen, watching as I took my first bite. My mouth was salivating as I placed the long-awaited hot buttered bread into my mouth. I chewed it a few times, promptly spat it out, and declared that I had been ripped off! It tasted nothing at all like bread. My family told me that I was overreacting. To prove it, they each tried the bread, and much to my satisfaction, they promptly spat it into the garbage. Needless to say, we were all sorely disappointed in the flavor and texture of the bread.

In order to save my pocketbook and in an attempt to eat gluten-free foods that were appealing, I developed a few gluten-free recipes that were actually palatable. Finally, after a month of gluten-free eating, unfortunately—or perhaps fortunately—there was still no change in my bowel habits. At the end of the month, the only positive outcome was increased empathy for people who suffer from gluten intolerance.

In all fairness, I must tell you that gluten-free products and mixes have come a long way since I first tried them. The flavor, texture, and availability have greatly improved, and even the price has decreased to about two and a half times the price of products containing gluten.

STOP TWO: IRRITABLE BOWEL SYNDROME

Irritable bowel syndrome (IBS) is also referred to as a "spastic colon" or an "irritable colon." I made a list of the symptoms of IBS and placing a check mark by each one I was experiencing. I no longer have the paper, but the list went something like this.

MY IBS SYMPTOMS

More common in women	I am a woman.
Diarrhea	Definitely not!
Constipation	YES!
Alternating diarrhea and constipation	No
Abdominal pain	Yes
Abdominal pain exacerbated by certain foods	I felt sicker after eating *anything*.
Pain over ileocecal valve; especially when area is palpated	Yes. Extremely tender.
Bloating	Yes
Flatulence	No
Loss of appetite	No
Depression	No
Anxiety	No
Normal endoscopy	Yes

Even though IBS didn't explain my migraines, belching, nausea, or insomnia, I became excited each time I had the sign or symptom listed. I thought if I had a diagnosis, I would be a step closer to finding a cure. I read that a diagnosis of IBS is based on patients having 60 percent or more of the signs and symptoms. I read further and discovered that there are two manifestations for IBS: diarrhea and constipation. It was reported that some physicians were having marginal success by treating patients with anti-depressant medications such as serotonin for the diarrhea form of IBS. Unfortunately no medications were available for individuals who suffer from the constipation variety of IBS. I might add that shortly after I ruled out IBS as a diagnosis, a new medication was approved; however, it was later removed from the market by the FDA.

Research articles also suggested that individuals suffering from either form of IBS should get adequate sleep, eliminate emotional stressors, reduce—if not eliminate—the consumption of stimulants, and as always, increase their intake of dietary fiber. Once again I was at a dead end because I didn't take stimulants. I wasn't stressed. And as far as fiber intake went, I was drinking fiber, taking fiber tablets, and eating fiber rich foods—there was no way I could add even more fiber to my diet unless I chopped down a tree and started gnawing it like a beaver. The time had come to investigate religious dietary doctrines.

CHAPTER THREE:

AND THE WISE AND
ANCIENT SPOKE

Throughout my life, I have had the pleasure of friendships, associations, and collaborative service opportunities involving wonderful people of Christian and non-Christian faiths. What I have learned from these choice people and opportunities is that there are universal concepts that are taught, supported, strived for, and eventually achieved, to one degree or another, among active members of most religions. If I were to jot down the more common universal religious concepts, my list would be as follows:

- Forgiveness
- Service
- Humility
- Love
- Selflessness
- Charity
- Emulation of a supreme being's qualities
  and characteristics
- Desire for unity with a supreme being

I believe these qualities, if practiced by an individual and his or her community, can lead to a state of nirvana, jannah, paradise, heaven, or a utopian society wherein there is eternal peace and rest.

I further believe that varying degrees of truth may be found in all religions. God loves mankind and desires that all should have truth, liberty of worship, physical health, enlightenment, blessings, and every success possible during their earthly sojourn.

I also believe that our earthly experience is meant to bring about personal growth and is superlatively designed to ensure that mankind succeeds! However, I must add that I also believe that man has an innate desire to experience pleasure over pain, to prefer ease over sacrifice, and to enjoy carnality over righteousness. Men and women often make quick, convenient, and hedonistic choices, thereby spurning God-given eternal truths that ensure health, joy, enlightenment, and both earthly and eternal success. Because all choices have positive or negative consequences associated with them, those who succumb to carnal desires eventually face inescapable negative consequences, which may include addiction, sexually transmitted diseases, financial ruin, unwanted pregnancies, loss of relationships, loss of health, and, most tragic of all, a loss of self-esteem.

I was fortunate to have been born of parents who encouraged me to investigate many religions during my youth. So, as an adult, it was natural for me to investigate many religions in an attempt to find a solution for my physical condition. I am grateful that I gained an appreciation for the truths found within these religions at a young age.

STOP THREE: CHRISTIANITY, THE HOLY BIBLE, AND DIETARY GUIDELINES

I am aware that there are many Christian and non-Christian religions throughout the world that do not, for a multitude of reasons, reference the King James Version (KJV) of the Holy Bible. Suffice to say, there are many translations of the Holy Bible, and each translation has its critics. However, I used the KJV in my research.

The Holy Bible has many verses addressing food; for example, biblical foods eaten (1 Samuel 17:18; 2 Samuel 17:13–29; Daniel 1:12–15; Ezekiel 4:9), the harmful nature of wine (Proverbs 23:30; Romans 14:21), and stories of miracles involving food (2 Kings 4; Matthew 14 and 15). However, if you are looking for *specific* dietary laws, which I was, you should read the first five books of the Old Testament.

GENESIS

Moses, an Old Testament prophet, wrote in Genesis 1:29 that mankind should eat, "Every herb bearing seed . . . and every tree in which is the fruit of a tree yielding seed." I found the word, "herb" to be puzzling. When I think of an herb, I think of a plant that doesn't have a woody trunk or branches and that provides flavor to foods or medicinal benefits to man through its roots, leaves, or seeds. Certainly, God did not intend for mankind's diet to consist entirely of herbs such as basil and cilantro and fruits from trees. What did the word "herb" mean in biblical times? I turned to the Latter-day Saint edition of the Holy Bible's topical guide and read the scriptural references for "herb." I discovered that in the Bible, herbs can be grains and vegetables (Genesis 3:18–19 and Deuteronomy 11:10). In Matthew 13 and Mark 4, we read the "Parable of the Mustard Seed," and surprisingly, this expansive tree is referred to as an herb in verse 32 of both accounts: "But when it is grown, *it is the greatest among herbs*." So much for my definition of an herb not having a woody trunk or branches.

Was Moses suggesting that mankind should be vegetarian? This was difficult for me to accept, especially after my personal experiences with a vegan diet in years past. Further readings revealed that mankind was allowed to eat meat. "Every moving thing that liveth shall be meat for you; even as the green herb have I given you all things" (Genesis 9:3). Moses also recorded God's caution not to drink animal blood: "But flesh with the life thereof, which is the blood thereof, shall ye not eat" (v. 4). As I read further in Genesis, I discovered that the prophet Noah was a farmer who raised livestock and had a vineyard (Genesis 9:20). Abraham offered bread, beef, butter, and milk to holy men (Genesis 18:6–8).

In addition to eating vegetables, fruits, grains, animal flesh, milk, and butter, I read that lentils, honey, spices, and nuts were consumed in biblical times as well. "Then Jacob gave Esau bread and pottage of lentils; and he did eat and drink"(Genesis 25:34). Food gifts are also noted in the Holy Bible: "Take of the best fruits of the land in your vessels, and carry down the man a present, a little balm, and a little honey, spices, and myrrh, nuts and almonds" (Genesis 43:11).

As I pondered the above scriptures and read further, two dietary trends became apparent. The first is that a typical meal in biblical times appears to have been largely grain- and vegetable-based and supplemented with occasional servings of fish, fowl, and meat. For example: Jacob's lentil stew and bread (Genesis 25:34); Ziba and his offering to King David (2 Samuel 16:1); Daniel and his companions requesting to eat pulse (Daniel 1:12–14); the man from Baal-shalisha who gave barley loaves and corn to feed the people (2 Kings 4:42); and Jesus' miracles feeding large numbers of people with a few loaves of bread and a few fish (Matthew 14:16–21; 15:32–37; and John 21:9).

The second trend was that meat (excluding fish), butter, and honey, were luxury foods that were eaten sparingly. Perhaps these foods were reserved for celebrations such as was written in the parable of the Return of the Prodigal Son (Luke 15:23); given to honored guests as demonstrated by Abraham feeding the holy men (Genesis 18:7); or given as gifts to prominent individuals as illustrated by Israel's food gift to Joseph (Genesis 43:11) and Abigail's, Shobbi's, Machir's, and Barzillia's food gifts to King David (1 Samuel 25:18; 2 Samuel 17: 28–29).

As a side note to those who may not be familiar with the writing styles found in the Holy Bible, authors of the Holy Bible often substituted the word "meat" for "food," much like they used the word herb to mean an actual herb, grains, or vegetables. A good example of this is when the apostle Paul wrote, "Esau who for one morsel of meat sold his birth right" (Hebrews 12:16); yet, one may read in Genesis 25:34 that Esau was not actually given meat but lentils and bread in exchange for his birthright.

EXODUS AND NUMBERS

Exodus and Numbers contained very little dietary information beyond the dietary restrictions of a Nazarite (Numbers 6:3–4, 20), foods reminiscent of that which was eaten while the Israelites were held captive in Egypt (Numbers 11:5), and foods that were brought back to Moses from the fertile and prosperous land of Canaan by Moses' scouts (Numbers 13:23, 27).

LEVITICUS AND DEUTERONOMY

You may recall that many Christian faiths (Eastern Orthodox, Greek Orthodox, Roman Catholic, and Seventh-day Adventist) as well as non-Christian, practicing Jews, base their dietary customs on the teachings found in the books of Leviticus and Deuteronomy. In the interest of brevity, the following table will summarize the dietary doctrine I found in these books.

LEVITICUS AND DEUTERONOMY DIETARY DOCTRINE

Restricted Animal-based Foods	Scriptural Reference
Blood	Leviticus 3:17, 7:26 Deuteronomy 12:16, 23
Foods that are offerings or tithing to God	Deuteronomy 12:17
Animal Fat	Leviticus 3:17, 7:23
Wine and strong drink	Leviticus 10:9
Camel, coney, hare, horse, and swine meat	Leviticus 11:4–7 Deuteronomy 14:7–8
Fish without fins and scales (catfish, eel, shark, shrimp, clam, crab, mussels, lobster, oysters, and so forth)	Leviticus 11:10 Deuteronomy 14:10
Eagle, ossifrage, osprey, vulture, kite, raven, owl, night hawk, cuckow, hawk, little owl, cormorant, great owl, swan, pelican, eagle, stork, heron, lapwing, bat, and fowls that creep on all fours.	Leviticus 11:13–20 Deuteronomy 14:12–19
Animals that go on paws on all fours (bear, raccoon, sloth)	Leviticus 11:27
Weasel, mouse, and tortoise	Leviticus 11:29
Ferret, chameleon, lizard, snail, and mole	Leviticus 11:30
Any carrion (dead animals) such as road kill	Leviticus 11:39 Deuteronomy 14:21
Creeping things (snakes, lizards, centipedes)	Leviticus 11:41–42

LEVITICUS AND DEUTERONOMY DIETARY DOCTRINE

Approved Animal-based Foods	Scriptural Reference
Animals with a parted hoof, cloven footed, and chews a cud (oxen, sheep, goat, hart, roebuck, fallow deer, pygarg, chamois, venison, elk, and antelope)	Leviticus 11:3 Deuteronomy 14:4–6
Fish with fins and scales such as trout, salmon, bass, halibut and so forth.	Leviticus 11:9 Deuteronomy 14:9
Locusts, bald locust, beetle, and grasshopper	Leviticus 11:22
All fowl (chickens, geese, turkey, ducks, and doves) except those mentioned as unclean in Leviticus 11:13–20 and Deuteronomy 14:12–19)	Deuteronomy 14:11, 20

It is surprising how your memory immediately improves, even though you don't prescribe to these dietary laws, when you realize you've broken commandments found in the Holy Bible, and I am not talking about my occasional eating of shrimp, crab, or rabbit. I am talking about a dietary violation that would be considered heinous by those who follow the dietary laws found in Leviticus and Deuteronomy.

Many years ago, we dined with some guests from China. My husband, Trent, requested our new friends to order their favorite homeland dishes, so they ordered chicken feet. I must admit that although there wasn't much meat, the sauce was absolutely delicious.

Our guests also ordered something that was a dull red color and had the consistency of thick gelatin. They said that this dish is known for improving the health of one's liver; however, they refused to tell us what it was until after we had tried it. Trent refused to eat it. I was game, but I should have known better when their children were wide-eyed and giggling.

Wanting to be a good sport, I took a spoonful and discovered that it tasted like liver. Liver is okay; however, I am not a gelatin eater, and as such, I had a difficult time swallowing the mystery food. Our friends laughed and shared the main ingredient of the mystery dish. It was congealed pig's blood. It took all I had to smile, laugh, and not vomit right then and there. Looking back, I treasure the memory, although I now realize that I managed to break two dietary commandments from the books of Leviticus and Deuteronomy in one bite!

Fasting—abstaining from food and water for a given period of time—was a common practice in biblical times. The length of a fast ranged from a day to 40 days (2 Samuel 12:16, Acts 27:33, Deuteronomy 9:9, Matthew 4:2, and Luke 4:2). Reasons for fasting varied greatly: King David fasted for his sick son (2 Samuel 12:16); King Darius fasted for the welfare of Daniel when he was cast into the lions den (Daniel 6:18); individuals and communities fasted for heavenly guidance, deliverance, and community protection (Ezra 8:23; 1 Kings 21:9; 2 Chronicles 20:3; Nehemiah 1:4; Esther 4:16, and Daniel 9:3).

There are two Christian religions I would like to discuss that believe in the Holy Bible and are also known for strict religious dietary guidelines: The Church of Jesus Christ of Latter-Day Saints and the Seventh-day Adventist Church.

THE CHURCH OF JESUS CHRIST OF LATTER-DAY SAINTS

The Church of Jesus Christ of Latter-day Saints, like other Christian religions, believes the King James Version of the Holy Bible is scripture. They also utilize additional sets of scripture called the Book of Mormon, the Doctrine and Covenants, and the Pearl of Great Price. Section 89 of the Doctrine and Covenants discusses diet in detail. Section 89 is also known as the Word of Wisdom, which members of the Church believe was received by revelation from the Lord to the Prophet Joseph Smith.

The Word of Wisdom categorizes food into three groups: foods that are healthful, foods that should be limited, and foods that are harmful. Healthful foods include vegetables, fruits, seeds, grains, legumes, and beans. The Doctrine and Covenants' scriptural passages are very broad, but the message is clear:

> And again, verily I say unto you, all wholesome herbs God hath
> ordained for the constitution, nature, and use of man. Every herb in

the season thereof, and every fruit in the season thereof; all these to be used with prudence and thanksgiving.

All grain is ordained for the use of man and of beasts, to be the staff of life, not only for man but for the beasts of the field, and the fowls of heaven, and all wild animals that run or creep on the earth; All grain is good for the food of man; as also the fruit of the vine; that which yieldeth fruit, whether in the ground or above the ground. Nevertheless, wheat for man, and corn for the ox, and oats for the horse, and rye for the fowls and for swine, and for all beasts of the field, and barley for all useful animals, and for mild drinks, as also other grain. (D&C 89:10–11, 14–17)

The Word of Wisdom teaches that mankind may eat meat; however, there are restrictions. "Yea, flesh also of beasts and of the fowls of the air, I, the Lord, have ordained for the use of man with thanksgiving; nevertheless they are to be used sparingly; And it is pleasing unto me that they should not be used, only in times of winter, or of cold, or famine" (D&C 89:12–13).

The foods that are considered harmful for mankind are wine, strong drink or alcohol, hot drinks, and tobacco. It should be noted that modern-day LDS prophets have interpreted "hot drinks" (D&C 89:5–9) to include coffee and tea.

Fasting is part of LDS doctrine as well. LDS members fast on the first Sunday of every month for two consecutive meals. There are many scriptural passages in Latter-day Saint religious texts that support the practice of fasting. Earlier I briefly explored Bible passages that detailed food and fasting guidelines for Christians, and in closing, I would like to share with you some of the LDS modern scriptural passages focusing on fasting that I found insightful and engaging. From the Book of Mormon: "Nevertheless they did fast and pray oft, and did wax stronger and stronger in their humility and firmer and firmer in the faith of Christ, unto the filling their souls with joy and consolation, yea, even to the purifying and the sanctification of their hearts, which sanctification cometh because of their yielding their hearts unto God" (Helaman 3:35). From the Doctrine and Covenants: "Verily, this is fasting and prayer, or in other words, rejoicing and prayer" (D&C 59:14). And lastly, my favorite passage, "Organize yourselves; prepare every needful thing; and establish a house, even a house of prayer, a house of fasting, a house of faith, a house of learning, a house of glory, a house of order, a house of God" (D&C 88:119).

SEVENTH-DAY ADVENTISTS

Seventh-day Adventist doctrine is based on the Holy Bible. Through the years, the Seventh-day Adventist Church has referenced multiple versions of the Holy Bible. I chose to study the Seventh-day Adventist Church Manual and referenced texts—the General Conference Position Statements and Guidelines for Dietary Doctrine.

Having never studied Seventh-day Adventist doctrine before, I decided to begin with the Seventh-day Adventist Church Manual. In the section on fundamental beliefs of Seventh-day Adventists, I read a beautiful passage containing holistic counsel, which, if followed, will lead to a Christlike state. Within this passage, followers are reminded that their bodies are temples of the Holy Spirit and as such, they should be cared for intelligently. I pondered the word intelligence, and the following words came to mind: wisdom, knowledge, discernment, analytical ability, and most important, application of knowledge to benefit yourself and others. I could have jumped with joy after reading this passage. To me, it bore witness that my quest for health could be obtained through intelligently evaluating religious dietary doctrines and scientific literature!

Further into the passage, I read the following: "Along with adequate exercise and rest, we are to adopt the most healthful diet possible and abstain from the unclean foods identified in the scriptures. Since alcoholic beverages, tobacco, and the irresponsible use of drugs and narcotics are harmful to our bodies, we are to abstain from them as well."

In support of these beliefs, the Seventh-day Adventists have instituted a Health Ministries Department, which has the "moral obligation" and charge of ministering to the ill, preventing disease, and providing health education. Reading the words "moral obligation" was powerful for me. I couldn't agree more; having a masters degree and a PhD(c) in public health, these words are dear to my heart. In my opinion, all of mankind has a moral obligation to come to the aid of all of the earth's inhabitants.

As I read further, I stood corrected in an erroneous belief that members of the Seventh-day Adventist faith are required to become vegetarian. "Where possible, members shall be encouraged to follow a primarily vegetarian diet." More specific dietary guidelines can be found in the section of the Church Manual on Health and Temperance:

> Health is promoted by an intelligent observance of the hygienic principles having to do with pure air, ventilation, suitable clothing, cleanliness, proper exercise and recreation, adequate sleep and rest, and an adequate, wholesome diet. God has furnished man with a liberal variety of foods sufficient to satisfy every dietary need. Fruits, grains, nuts, and vegetables prepared in simple ways "make, with milk or cream, the most healthful diet."

In addition to the Church Manual, General Conference Statements, and Guidelines for Dietary Doctrine, I found the Seventh-day Adventist Dietetic Association (http://www.sdada.org). This association's purpose is to provide healthful living through a plant-based diet. I would recommend vegetarians of any faith to take advantage of the information provided by this site. You will find a vegetarian food pyramid, health tips on foods and exercise, helps for menu planning, and commercial links for vegetarian products and information.

Perhaps the most beneficial section for me was the Seventh-day Adventist Position Statement on Vegetarian Diets, which nicely summarized the diet recommended by the General Conference of the Seventh-day Adventist's Nutrition Council (GCNC):

> The GCNC recommends that all meat, fish, and fowl be eliminated from the diet and the use of egg yolks be limited to three or less per week. Foods of animal origin are no longer viewed as dominant items in a healthy diet. The Adventist Health Study clearly reveals a significant advantage for those who choose a meat-free, plant-based diet over those who select primarily a meat-based diet.
>
> The GCNC recommends the generous use of whole grains, vegetables and fruits; and a moderate use of low fat dairy products (or nutritional equivalent alternatives), legumes, and nuts; a very limited use of foods high in saturated fat, cholesterol, sugar, and salt; abstinence from tobacco, alcohol, and coffee, tea, and other caffeinated beverages.

STOP FOUR: NON-CHRISTIAN RELIGIONS' FASTING AND DIETARY GUIDELINES

BUDDHISM

I have always considered Buddhism to be a religion; however, after reading articles on Buddhist principles, I realized that I was once again guilty of ignorance. Buddhism is not a religion, but more of a lifestyle choice based on the philosophies of Buddha. I say that Buddhism is not a religion because Buddhism does not require the worshipping of deity. In fact, much to my surprise, Buddhist followers do not even worship Buddha; they bow in an effort to express respect and humble gratitude to Buddha for sharing his enlightening principles with others.

I could have spent years reading and studying all of the literature available on Buddhism. Because my primary interest was in dietary laws, I spent several days reading about Buddhism in general and then delved into Buddhism's dietary guidelines. I learned that certain sects of Buddhists are prohibited from consuming meat, alcohol, and drugs. Although I am cognizant of the reality that one Christian religion may not follow religious doctrine to the same degree of rigor as another Christian religion, I was flabbergasted at my ignorance when I read that there are varying degrees of dietary strictness within each Buddhist sect. Why was I shocked to learn this? Well, let's put it this way. If I were on a game show and asked if all Buddhists are vegetarians, I would have emphatically answered, "Yes! All Buddhists are vegetarians due to the first Moral Precept, which states that one should not kill or harm living things." You would then hear a loud long buzzer, which would signal that I was *wrong!* Buddhists may or may not eat meat. Choosing to eat meat does not impact one's path to nirvana; however, participation in the act of slaughtering animals does delay progression.

Many Buddhists refrain from eating the Five Pungent Spices: onions, garlic, scallions, chives, and leeks. According to the Shurangama Sutra, these spices should not be eaten because they increase one's sexual desire or anger and recoil good Gods while beckoning hungry ghosts and demons.

Conceivably, the timeliest Buddhist principles in terms of our present-day environmental concerns are Buddha's Five Contemplations While Eating. In the Five Contemplations While Eating, Buddha shares his thoughts before selecting and eating food:

1. I think about where the food came from and the amount of work necessary to grow the food, transport it, prepare and cook it and bring it to the table.
2. I contemplate my own virtuous nature. Is it sufficient to merit receiving the food as offering?
3. I guard my mind against transgression, the principal ones being greed and so forth.
4. I realize that food is a wholesome medicine that heals the sufferings of the body.
5. I should receive the food offerings only for the sake of realizing the Way.

These profound words of wisdom provided me with a valuable opportunity to evaluate my personal food selection. Here are six thoughts that came to mind as I reflected on the Five Contemplations While Eating.

1. As I look at the beautifully displayed meat, dairy, fish, fruits, and vegetables in the grocery store, do I really stop and think about what goes into raising, preparing, and shipping the foods I choose to purchase and eat?
2. Do I express sincere gratitude for the animals, fruits, vegetables, and water that God has placed on the planet for the health and benefit of mankind?
3. On a daily basis, do I experience heartfelt thankfulness for the lives of the plants and animals that were sacrificed so that I might live?
4. Am I eating to live or living to eat? In other words, do I consider my personal food choices in terms of necessity versus gluttony?
5. Are my food choices exploiting the earth's natural resources for unnecessary personal gratification? In other words, how are my food choices affecting fisheries', farmers', ranchers', and businesses' production decisions? How are economically based food production decisions affecting the earth's delicately balanced ecosystem?

6. Am I making intelligent food choices or impulsive ones? Am I choosing to eat whatever my body is craving or what is readily available?

I truly believe that if people would consciously evaluate their food demands based on the principles of the Five Contemplations While Eating, individual health would improve, civilization's destructive impact on the earth would lessen, the earth's environmental quality would recover, and the earth's productivity would increase. After reading and pondering Buddha's Five Contemplations While Eating, I will be, from this point forward, filled with more introspection, gratitude, and reverence for the wondrous foods available to mankind. Thank you, Buddha, for sharing. You have truly enlightened my mind regarding the blessedness of food.

HINDUISM

Hindus classify food into three categories: *sattvic, rajasic,* and *tamasic. Sattvic* foods are considered to be of the purest or highest order. These foods include fresh fruits, raw or slightly cooked vegetables, herbs, whole grains, legumes, nuts, seeds, butter, cheese, honey, and milk. *Rajasic* foods are foods that induce passion and are less desirable than *sattvic* foods. *Rajasic* foods include onions, garlic, coffee, black tea, sugar-laden foods, chocolate, spicy and salted food, and tobacco. *Tamasic* foods are the least desirable for the body and should be avoided. These foods include meat; fish; fowl; eggs; mushrooms; vinegar; any fried, burned, reheated, or fermented foods; as well as any form of alcohol or drugs.

Why are Hindus encouraged not to eat meat? I also wondered where I could find a scriptural reference to the *sattvic, rajasic,* and *tamasic* foods. During my research of sacred Hindu texts, I discovered that there are many English translations of Hindu texts on the Internet, so I decided to read and compare the styles of a few translations until I found one that resonated with me. Before too long, I developed a fondness toward a particular translator's style.

Once I had selected the translated version of the Hindu text that I wanted to read, I settled in at my desk for an enjoyable day of reading. As I read these enriching stories, words of wisdom, poems, and hymns, I escaped into another world. Time passed quickly, and soon my children were home from school, and my husband was home from work. Pillow talk with my husband at night centered on the verses I had read that day and how they supported, added a new dimension to, or differed from our beliefs. My husband was so interested that he asked me to record the passages and chapters that had the highest impact on me so that he could more fully share my experience. It was a beneficial and engaging exercise, to say the least. Perhaps it was the translation that I chose to read, or maybe it was that the messages were in story form. Whatever it was, the concepts were clear, poignant, and multidimensional.

Some sacred Hindu texts, such as the *Bhagavad-Gita*, are divided into chapters and verses, like the Christian Bible. Other sacred texts are divided into *cantos,* or long poems or hymns. When attempting to locate a particular passage, the first number in the reference is the specific canto, the following number is the chapter within the canto, and the last number is the quoted text.

The Bhagavad-Gita 17:7–10 and associated Vaisnava Sampra-dayas commentaries contain passages that categorize foods into *sattvic, rajasic,* and *tamasic* levels. Hindus may choose to fast as an offering of worship (4:29), and they are also encouraged to eat moderately (18:51–53). You may be surprised to learn that not all Hindus are vegetarians. Abstaining from meat is encouraged; however, it is not considered sinful behavior to eat meat (5:56).

In my estimation, the Hindu law of *Ahinsa,* or non-injury, is one of the most powerful Hindu laws in support of vegetarianism. This law applies not only to humans but also to all living animals. There are literally hundreds of scriptures testifying of *Ahinsa* and the blessings that follow through obedience. Some of the more commonly cited verses can be read in the *Vedas.* Here are a few of my personal favorites: "By not killing any living being, one becomes fit for salvation" (6.60). "Those noble souls who practice meditation and other yogic ways, who are ever careful about all beings, who protect all animals, are the ones who are actually serious about spiritual practices" (19.48.5). "One should be considered dear, even by the animal kingdom" (17.1.4). "Those who have no knowledge of these facts and very unholy presumptuously consider themselves saintly, do harm to innocently trusting animals; upon leaving their bodies will those animals eat them" (11.5.14). "What is virtue? 'Tis not to kill, for killing causes every ill" (321).

JUDAISM

The Judaic dietary laws, or *kashrut*, are recorded in the Holy Torah as well as the Holy Talmud. Many Christians may say that they have never read the Holy Torah. This is not entirely correct. The first five books of the Holy Bible—Genesis, Exodus, Leviticus, Numbers, and Deuteronomy— are the Holy Torah. As I read the scriptures, I was so excited to tell my husband, "Trent, do you realize that the Torah is one of the first public health texts?" Trent just looked at me and said, "What do you mean? It's the first five books of the Bible, isn't it?" I explained that the Holy Torah was, and still is, a sacred text that addresses public health and safety through specific hygiene and dietary laws, which, if followed, will decrease the risks of disease and death. The Torah teaches principles of sanitation, infection control, disease prevention, and health education. Don't tell my public health students this, but every semester, I toy with the idea of adding an assignment of reading the Holy Torah and the Holy Bible and requiring them to address the ancient wisdoms in every verse that promotes public health and safety.

Dietary laws can be found in the books of Torat Kohanim (Leviticus) and Devarim (Deuteronomy). A brief summary of these laws is provided in the table below. A smattering of additional dietary and food preparation methods can be found throughout the Torah.

TORAT KOHANIM (LEVITICUS) AND DEVARIM (DEUTERONOMY) DIETARY DOCTRINE

Restricted Animal-based Foods	Scriptural Reference
Blood	Leviticus 3:17, 7:26 Deuteronomy 12:16, 23
Foods that are offerings or tithing to God	Deuteronomy 12:17
Animal Fat	Leviticus 3:17, 7:23
Wine and Strong Drink	Leviticus 10:9

Restricted Animal-based Foods	Scriptural Reference
Camel, coney, hare, horse, and swine meat	Leviticus 11:4–7 Deuteronomy 14:7–8
Fish without fins and scales (catfish, eel, shark, shrimp, clam, crab, mussels, lobster, oysters, and so on)	Leviticus 11:10 Deuteronomy 14:10
Eagle, ossifrage, osprey, vulture, kite, raven, owl, night hawk, cuckow, hawk, little owl, cormorant, great owl, swan, pelican, gier eagle, stork, heron, lapwing, bat and fowls that creep on all fours.	Leviticus 11:13–20 Deuteronomy 14:12–19
Animals which go on paws on all fours (bear, raccoon, sloth)	Leviticus 11:27
Weasel, mouse, and tortoise	Leviticus 11:29
Ferret, chameleon, lizard, snail, and mole	Leviticus 11:30
Any carrion (dead animals such as road kill)	Leviticus 11:39 Deuteronomy 14:21
Creeping things (snakes, lizards, centipedes)	Leviticus 11:41–42
Approved Animal-based Foods	Scriptural Reference
Animals with a parted hoof, cloven footed, and chews a cud (ox, sheep, goat, hart, roebuck, fallow deer, pygarg, chamois, venison, elk, and antelope)	Leviticus 11:3 Deuteronomy 14:4–6
Fish with fins and scales (trout, salmon, bass, halibut and so on)	Leviticus 11:9 Deuteronomy 14:9
Locusts, bald locusts, beetles, and grasshoppers.	Leviticus 11:22
All fowl (chickens, geese, turkey, ducks, and doves) except those mentioned as unclean in Leviticus 11:13–20 and Deuteronomy 14:12–19)	Deuteronomy 14:11, 20

ISLAM

I was surprised to discover that an Islamic diet is not as restrictive as I had thought. Foods that are *Halal* are good for the body and should be eaten regularly. These include milk, honey, fish with scales, plants that are non-addictive and do not contain intoxicants, grains, vegetables and fruits, legumes, nuts, seeds, and beans. Muslims can eat meat from cattle, sheep, deer, goats, moose, chickens, turkey, ducks, geese, and so on, if slaughtered according to Islamic customs.

Foods that are classified as *Haraam* are foods that should not be eaten. These include animals improperly slaughtered according to Islamic customs, pork and pork by-products, horse, donkey, or mule, meat-eating animals, birds of prey, any animal blood, rabbit, dogs, elephants, monkeys, and animals without ears. There appeared to be some disagreement among authors as to whether crustaceans and fish without scales should be eaten. Those that support eating these foods quote the Holy Qur'an, Abdullah Yusufali translation 35:12, which reads, "Nor are the two bodies of flowing water alike—the one palatable, sweet, and pleasant to drink, and the other, salt and bitter. Yet from each (kind of water) do ye eat flesh fresh and tender, and ye extract ornaments to wear; and thou seest the ships therein that plough the waves, that ye may seek (thus) of the Bounty of Allah that ye may be grateful."

Once I identified differences of opinion on eating certain sea creatures, I decided to explore the Holy Qur'an for myself, choosing to read the Abdullah Yusufali translation. The Holy Qur'an consists of 114 chapters, which are the recorded teachings of Allah. Allah is the deity worshipped by Muslims. When looking up a particular passage of interest, the first number references a specific chapter within the Holy Qur'an, and the next number is the verse within that chapter, much like a biblical citation. As is the case with many religious texts, there are many translations for the Holy Qur'an. In order to enjoy religious texts to their fullest extent, compare several translations until you find the one that is most meaningful to you.

My reading of the Holy Qur'an was very fruitful; I managed to identify specific verses that addressed dietary counsel from Allah. Though I identified four passages in the Holy Qur'an that described what foods are forbidden, or *Halaam* (2:173; 5:3; 6:145; 16:115), the following verses were most beneficial for me in understanding the concept of *Halaam* foods.

> Forbidden to you (for food) are: dead meat, blood, the flesh of swine, and that on which hath been invoked the name of other than Allah; that which hath been killed by strangling, or by a violent blow, or by a headlong fall, or by being gored to death; that which hath been (partly) eaten by a wild animal; unless ye are able to slaughter it (in due form); that which is sacrificed on stone (altars); (forbidden) also is the division (of meat) by raffling with arrows: that is impiety. This day have those who reject faith given up all hope of your religion: yet fear them not but fear Me. This day have I perfected your religion for you, completed My favour upon you, and have chosen for you Islam as your religion. But if any is forced by hunger, with no inclination to transgression, Allah is indeed Oft-forgiving, Most Merciful" (5:3).

In addition to identifying what should not be eaten, I found two beautiful verses that promote mankind eating God-given food as well as growing and eating fruits and vegetables. "O ye who believe! Eat of the good things that We have provided for you, and be grateful to Allah, if it is Him ye worship" (2:172). "It is He Who produceth gardens, with trellises and without, and dates, and tilth with produce of all kinds, and olives and pomegranates, similar (in kind) and different (in variety): eat of their fruit in their season, but render the dues that are proper on the day that the harvest is gathered. But waste not by excess: for Allah loveth not the wasters" (6:141).

And lastly, I was able to locate a warning from Allah that addresses the harmful consequences that can be associated with alcohol. "Satan's plan is (but) to excite enmity and hatred between you, with intoxicants and gambling, and hinder you from the remembrance of Allah, and from prayer: will ye not then abstain?" (5:91).

Muslims practice a yearly fast called Ramadan, which lasts under most circumstances for twenty-nine days. During Ramadan, Muslims refrain from consuming food and fluids from sunrise to sunset. Not all Muslims are required to fast. Pregnant women, nursing mothers, and young children are exempt from fasting as well as people who are traveling (2:183–185).

In addition to observing Ramadan, Muslims may also fast to

become closer to Allah, to receive wisdom and blessings, and to show penitence (2:196; 5:89; 5:95; 33:35; 66:5). For further information regarding the occasions and circumstances in which Muslims fast, refer to the Hadith, a collection of ancient prophetic words and traditions of the revered Islamic prophet Muhammad. The prophet Muhammad often fasted and encouraged others to fast, as illustrated by hundreds of citations found in the Hadith collections.

CHAPTER FOUR:

TESTING AND
PROVING TRUTH

STOP FIVE: SCIENTIFIC VALIDATION OF THE BENEFITS OF RELIGIOUS DIETARY DOCTRINE

Before I discuss researching scientific studies examining the health and longevity of members of religious sects, I want to examine the validity of my doctor-prescribed treatment of constipation, namely, increased water intake, exercise, and above all, increased fiber intake. I found several peer-reviewed articles to help me in this endeavor.

Review articles published in scholarly journals evaluate and summarize peer-reviewed research papers on a given topic. Review articles are susceptible to shortcomings such as publication bias, which can occur when the hypothesis is rejected. In other words, more often than not, research has a better chance of being published if the intervention of a product, practice, or treatment leads to positive results, especially if the research is being financially supported by a product manufacturer. On the other hand, research that demonstrates little difference of a particular intervention is less likely to become published.

Another limitation of review articles is the language barrier. The reader may not read past the article's abstract if the article is not written in his known language(s). Lastly, review papers' conclusions are based on the aggregate of studies reviewed; therefore, the review article's conclusions may be weak or erroneous if the individual studies contain design or methodological flaws. In conclusion, always be cautious and critically aware of what you are reading.

I was pleased to find review articles by Felix Leung and Muller-Lissner et al. because both review papers pointed out that there is a dearth of evidence-based research on the cause of constipation. After drinking an entire ocean of water, eating a forest of fiber, and exercising more than I ever wanted to without any change in my condition, I finally felt validated!

Both articles confirmed that increasing water intake may aid in constipation relief if the patient is dehydrated. Dietary fiber, on the other hand, has been shown to increase constipation in some study participants and decrease constipation in others. The only constipation treatment that appeared to contribute to a modest improvement in constipation was physical activity. After reading this review, I felt vindicated! It also piqued my interest in researching other dietary aspects of constipation.

EVIDENCE-BASED FINDINGS FOR RELIGIOUS DIETARY DOCTRINE

Before launching into the scientific evidence, I must once again extend a word of caution to readers. When interpreting study results, the reader must be aware of an epidemiologic term called "confounding." A confounder is any category or trait of study participants that is associated with a particular outcome that may lead to an imprecise interpretation of study results. For example: a scientist conducts a study on the causes of lung cancer. She asks the participants about their lives and determines that coffee drinkers experience a higher rate of lung cancer. Does drinking coffee really cause a greater risk of lung cancer or is it that the consumption of coffee is more prevalent among tobacco smokers? The answer is easily determined by comparing the rate of lung cancer among non-smoking coffee drinkers and smoking coffee drinkers. We would discover that tobacco usage or being exposed to secondary smoke while drinking coffee is associated with an increased risk of lung cancer. As such, the associated behavior of coffee drinking is a confounder.

Most of the religions I explored proscribe alcohol and tobacco usage. This means that if the scientists conducting studies have not controlled for the influence of alcohol and tobacco, the abstinence from alcohol and tobacco may actually be the behavior that is affecting the positive outcome on health rather than the religious diet and is therefore a confounder.

RELIGIOUS SCIENTIFIC STUDIES

THE CHURCH OF JESUS CHRIST OF LATTER-DAY SAINTS

Search words:	Website Hits
"LDS morbidity"	0 articles
"Mormon and longevity"	0 articles
"Mormon morbidity"	67 articles
"Mormon mortality"	29 articles
"Mormon health"	42 articles
"Mormon and fasting"	1 article

Though there were many articles examining various health issues of LDS church members, I could not identify an article that specifically addressed the LDS diet found in section 89 of the Doctrine and Covenants. However, I did find several studies that established that LDS members who practice abstinence from alcohol and tobacco have lower cancer and death rates than the general population. In addition to these studies, I found a very interesting study that identified a positive relationship between regular fasting and a decrease in the incidence of coronary heart disease and diabetes among LDS members.

BUDDHISM

Search words	Website Hits
"Buddhist and mortality"	7 articles, none examining diet
"Buddhist and morbidity"	17 articles, one examining diet
"Buddhists and health"	32 articles, none examining diet
"Buddhist and fasting"	1 article

I was surprised at the dearth of scientific research specifically examining Buddhist dietary health. After thinking about this odd lack of information, it became apparent that I had not selected the

correct search words. If 90 percent or more of a country is a specific religion or lifestyle, would scientists include the name of the
predominate "religion" in their studies? Probably not. Therefore, I
searched using "Asian diet" and immediately identified 1,581 articles! Obviously I needed to refine the rest of my search terms. A
myriad of research has been conducted regarding the typical Asian
vegetarian diet and its associated benefits, which include a decrease
in risk of heart disease, diabetes, and cancer.

ISLAM

I searched www.pubmed.gov, the official website of the National Institutes of Health (NIH) using the following words, "Muslim diet and
mortality, morbidity, longevity, fasting, and Ramadan." Over 1,900
articles examined the practice of intermittent prolonged fasting during
Ramadan. Some of the studies examined stroke, heart disease, asthma
attacks, emergency room visits, maternal and neonatal health, physical activity, as well as numerous other diseases and biological systems
for untoward effects associated with Ramadan. After a good deal of
reading, I came to the same conclusion as the vast majority of authors:
prolonged intermittent fasting does not permanently nor significantly
alter one's health, nor does it increase the risk for or exacerbation of
diseases, with the exception of diabetes, which requires additional
education and modification of daily medications.

HINDUISM

Search words: "Hinduism and diet, mortality, morbidity, and
health" revealed only three pertinent articles that identified relationships between a vegetarian diet and an increased risk of tuberculosis, Cobalamin (B12) deficiencies, and megaloblastic anemia
among Hindu Asians. I conducted a cursory literature review using
the words "Asian Indian" and "vegetarian" and found studies that
substantiated the nutritional deficiencies associated with vegetarian
diets and increased risks for megaloblastic anemia, tuberculosis, and
deficiencies of vitamins B6, B12, and D.

Similar to my issue with searching for Buddhism, I found little
research using the word "Hindu" or "Hinduism," so I decided to
include the words "Asian Indian" and "vegetarian diet" and was

rewarded with twenty-two articles. Unfortunately, I was unable to locate dietary studies involving Asian Indians or Hindus that did not focus on dietary deficiencies, diseases, and conditions as a result of a strict vegetarian diet and poverty. Poverty or socioeconomic status is typically a confounder.

Poverty for vegetarians and non-vegetarians alike limits the ability to purchase a variety of foods; this alone lends itself to suboptimal nutrition. There is also the issue of food availability in poorer communities. Do study participants from lower socioeconomic classes have the luxury of finding a well-stocked food market near their homes? Do they have the time, land, and means to farm a home-grown, well-balanced diet? If poorer communities in southern Asia are anything like poorer communities in the United States and other developed nations throughout the world, the answer is no. I am also fairly certain that few, if any, of the study participants who were considered poverty stricken ever attended nutrition classes or had access to a dietician. Therefore, I suggest that the dietary deficiencies described in the studies are not attributed so much to vegetarianism as to untoward elements of poverty.

To further support my belief, consider this 2009 statement on vegetarianism from the American Dietetic Association:

"It is the position of the American Dietetic Association that appropriately planned vegetarian diets, including total vegetarian or vegan diets, are healthful, nutritionally adequate, and may provide health benefits in the prevention and treatment of certain diseases. Well-planned vegetarian diets are appropriate for individuals during all stages of the life cycle, including pregnancy, lactation, infancy, childhood, and adolescence, and for athletes."

As I thought about these studies and identified their deficiencies, I recalled how my body would crave meat, milk, and eggs after about six months of eating a vegan diet. I never met with a dietician; I simply applied my rudimentary knowledge about vegetarianism, and within six months, I developed unbearable cravings for meat, milk, and eggs, all of which are natural food sources for B6, B12, and Vitamin D. Out of curiosity, I decided to explore what NIH had to say about vitamins B6, B12, and D deficiencies. After reading about dietary sources of vitamins B6, B12, and D and the signs, symptoms, and diseases associated with deficiencies of these vitamins, I have this word of advice: To ensure nutritional balance and optimal health, consult with a registered dietician before adopting a vegan diet.

SEVENTH-DAY ADVENTIST CHURCH

Hundreds of studies have examined the health of Seventh-day Adventist Church members who adhere to a lacto-ovo-vegetarian or a vegetarian diet. Studies have concluded that Seventh-day Adventists who chose a plant-based diet have less risk for developing certain cancers, obesity, heart disease, diabetes, and hypertension, and live longer than those who do not.

JUDAISM

Search words: "Torah, diet, longevity, health, and mortality"; "Judaism, health, and diet"; "Jewish, hypertension, cancer, stroke, and nutrition"; "Rosh Hashanah"; and "Public health, Torah, Talmud, halakha, and kashrut" did not reveal topically pertinent articles. I moved on to the effects of fasting and entered the search words, "Jewish fasting" and "Yom Kippur," which resulted in seventy-one hits.

Yom Kippur, the Day of Atonement, is a twenty-five-hour fasting period observed by faithful Jews. Of the seventy-one articles, two noted an increase in newborn deliveries within one day of Yom Kippur. A more recent article refuted this claim and stated that there was not a difference in birth rates. Additional articles discussed and evaluated the occurrence of the "Yom Kippur headache" and effective pharmacological remedies.

As I have mentioned earlier in the book, I am fascinated by public health and food-borne illnesses. The following are a few food-borne illnesses that would be curtailed by following wisdom found in the Holy Torah, which is also supported by scientific literature.

It is a good idea not to consume blood or raw meats because life-threatening pathogens can live in blood at various stages in their life cycles. The World Health Organization (WHO) reported that some fatalities from the Avian Influenza H5N1 may have been transmitted to humans by eating raw blood-based dishes (Leviticus 3:17; 7:26; and Deuteronomy 12:16, 23).

Disease/bacteria	Blood-based source	Biblical Reference
Toxocariasis	raw beef liver	n/a
Gnathostomiasis	raw fish or crustacean dishes	Leviticus 11:10, Deuteronomy 14:10
Trichinellosis	undercooked or raw horse	Leviticus 11:4–7 Deuteronomy 14:7–8
	bear	Leviticus 11:27
	seal	Leviticus 11:10, Deuteronomy 14:10
	walrus	Leviticus 11:10, Deuteronomy 14:10
	fox	Leviticus 11:27
	dog	Leviticus 11:27
	wolf	Leviticus 11:27
	pork	Leviticus 11:7
	wild cats such as cougar	Leviticus 11:27
Angiostrongyliasis	raw or undercooked prawns	Leviticus 11:10 Deuteronomy 14:10
	crab	Leviticus 11:10 Deuteronomy 14:10
	frogs and snails	Leviticus 11:30
Tape worms	undercooked beef.	
Vibrio arahaemolyticus infections and Norwalk viruses	undercooked oysters, clams, mussels, and scallops	Leviticus 11:10 Deuteronomy 14:10
Vibrio vulnificus	raw oysters	Leviticus 11:10, Deuteronomy 14:10.

As if you aren't already questioning ever eating food again, please keep in mind that the food-borne illnesses listed above are only a minute fraction of the many that plague mankind. There are two impressions that I hope you have gained from this extremely brief examination of food-borne illnesses and the Holy Torah. The first impression is that following the food laws in the Torah was and is protective against many food-borne pathogens. And second, if you are going to eat the forbidden flesh foods of the Torah, remember they need to be thoroughly cooked or your risk for food-borne illnesses will increase.

For more information on food safety, food borne illnesses, current outbreaks, and food recalls, I recommend the United States Food Safety website (foodsafety.gov)

STUDIES COMPARING DIFFERENT RELIGIONS' HEALTH IN THE AGGREGATE

I was only able to locate a few studies that compared the health status of members of differing faiths. It is interesting to note that most of the studies involved members of the Church of Jesus Christ of Latter-day Saints and Seventh-day Adventists. At first this appeared to be a peculiar oversight of other religions; however, after giving this situation thoughtful consideration, it is more than likely due to active Mormons and Adventists experiencing greater longevity and abstaining from alcohol, tobacco, and illicit drugs.

A study published in the American Journal of Clinical Nutrition examined the differences in blood pressures between LDS omnivores and Adventist vegetarians. Beilin discovered that Adventist vegetarians had less hypertension and overall lower blood pressure readings when compared with LDS omnivores. Beilin suggests differences in diets were a contributing factor.

Another study compared Mormons' and Adventists' incidence of cancer and life expectancy with that of citizens within the Federal Republic of Germany. Data demonstrated that LDS and Adventists had fewer deaths attributed to certain types of cancers, such as oral, lung, throat, colon, rectum, prostate, and cervical cancers. An unexpected finding identified by researchers was an increased rate of malignant melanoma, lymphoma, and myeloma among LDS members when compared to the German population.

The third study examined differences in cholesterol levels, blood pressure, and diabetes between Hispanic vegetarian Adventists and Catholic omnivores. The findings reported by Alexander et al. were in favor of a vegetarian diet, with Adventists demonstrating lower cholesterol values, lower blood pressure readings, and a lower risk for Type 2 diabetes.

The last study examined risk factors for heart disease such as cholesterol levels, blood pressure, smoking and so on between Thai-Muslims and Thai-Buddhists. Many of the cardiovascular risk factors were statistically insignificant between the two populations; however, Yipintsoi found that male Buddhists had higher high density lipo proteins (HDL, or good cholesterol) than male Muslims. Female Muslims had a higher prevalence of hypertension than female Buddhists.

CHAPTER FIVE:

FASTING— LESS IS MORE

STOP SIX: THE RETURN TRIP

Before I present the diet that I developed based on my findings, it seems fitting to discuss the absence of food in one's dietary regime, or in other words, the practice of fasting. All of the religions I studied fasted in one form or another. Fasting may be defined as an absence of some types of foods, such as during the Lent or Ekadashi; an absence of foods during religious holidays, for example Ramadan or Kavadi; abstinence from certain types of food on specific days of the week, such as no meat on Fridays for certain Catholic sects; abstinence from foods and fluids for a specified number of hours or days such as Ramadan for Muslims; or fasting on the first Sunday of the month and times of special need for members of the Church of Jesus Christ of Latter-Day Saints.

Reasons for fasting vary among religious sects from efforts to increase self-restraint (Qur'an 2:183), help the ill (2 Samuel 12:16), deliverance during times of war (2 Chronicles 20:3), or to receive a witness or knowledge (Alma 5:46).

Fasting is not advised for all people. For example, diabetics and hypoglycemics, young children, and pregnant or nursing women should not fast. I strongly encourage you to consult with your family physician to determine if your body can safely abstain from foods and fluids during periods of fasting.

Fasting was not a new concept to me. I was taught by my mother to fast once a month as part of my religious worship; however, my parents did not force me to fast. They gently reminded me that it was fast Sunday and casually asked if I wanted something for breakfast. There was no stern glance of disapproval or disparaging remark if I chose to eat breakfast. When I was twelve, I decided that I should begin fasting on a monthly basis. It was a horrible experience. By the time dinner was on the table, I had developed hunger pangs, a dry throat, a headache, and extreme irritability. My thoughts did not center on God, religion, or the person or situation I was fasting for; no, not at all. My thoughts centered on *food* and a nice tall drink of water! Needless to say, fasting was hit and miss during my youth.

During early adulthood, I attempted to fast not only for religious reasons but also in an attempt to gain bowel regularity. I speculated that my digestive tract was overwhelmed or overworked, causing severe constipation. Perhaps if I gave it a regular rest from foods and fluids, I would be able to eliminate waste on a daily basis. I wish I could tell you that fasting once a week helped me physically, but it didn't.

In 2001, I committed to fasting for religious reasons. I attempted fasting "cold turkey" from food and fluids for twelve hours at a time. Once again, I relived the memories of fasting from my childhood, only this time I wasn't edgy with my younger brother and parents; I was tense and irritable toward my husband and children. In my estimation, using a "cold turkey" approach to fasting did not bring a higher level of spirituality into our home and definitely did not bring me closer to developing God-like attributes. Because I believe that one must master his body before he can master his spirit, I earnestly desired to become successful at fasting.

Eventually I developed a strategy that helped me abstain from foods and fluids for twelve hours with ease. I figured that my irritability and illness during previous fasting experiences was because I didn't ease into fasting. So if I were to gradually increase the duration of my fasts, maybe I could limit any negative symptoms. If my hypothesis was right, I should theoretically be able to incrementally increase my the duration of my fasts and experience few if any symptoms during the process.

I committed to listening to my body's responses during fasting. My goal, at first, was to fast from after dinner to 10 a.m. the next morning. All went well with the exception of thirst. As my fast continued, my thirst grew, and my throat steadily became drier until I began coughing. It was after experiencing this that I decided to create personal rules expressly designed to enable me to succeed at fasting.

RULE 1: *DRINK A GLASS OF WATER IN THE MORNING IF NEEDED.*

The next time I chose to fast, I started my morning with a glass of water. This glass of water was what I needed; I wasn't uncomfortably parched as the morning progressed, and I successfully fasted until 10 a.m.

The next time I fasted, I increased my fast to noon. I was a little hungry, and so for the next few months, I didn't increase the length of my fasts past noon. I discovered a pattern over the months that followed. If I woke up hungry or feeling puny, I could not even fast until 10 a.m.

RULE 2: *IF I WAKE UP HUNGRY, FEELING PUNY, OR SICK, I WILL FAST ON ANOTHER DAY.*

The time came to increase my fast to 2 p.m. Fasting until 2 p.m. did not go as well as I had hoped. I was hungry, developed a slight headache, and thought more of food than I care to admit. I tried fasting until 2 p.m. for three or four months. Not much changed; nonetheless, I did notice something rather interesting. If I had eaten a moderately portioned meal the night before I started my fast, I could fast without difficulty. On the other hand, if I had eaten a full prime rib dinner the night prior to fasting, I would be abnormally hungry in the morning. I then found it nearly impossible to fast until 2 p.m. In reference to my experience, I was able to find one scientific article that examined types of meals eaten and ease of fasting. Blondheim et al. concluded that a low-protein, pre-fasting meal appears to increase the ease of fasting.

Here is what various religions have to say regarding overeating and fasting. In the Bhagavad-Gita 18:51–53, Hindu followers are told that by giving up sense objects and eating moderately, one can enter into a blissful state and communion with the Supreme Lord.

Saheeh al-Jaami found this prudent advice concerning gluttony in the Hadith collection, recorded by the Muslim scholar Muhammad al-Bukhari: "Man fills no vessel worse than his stomach. It is sufficient for the son of Adam to have a few mouthfuls to give him the strength he needs. If he has to fill his stomach, then let him leave one-third for food, one-third for drink and one-third for air" (Saheeh al-Jaami' 5,674).

In the Hadith, Muslims are taught that Allah's apostle said, "The food for two persons is sufficient for three, and the food of three persons is sufficient for four persons" (Volume 7, Book 65, Number 304). Furthermore, "By Him in Whose Hands my soul is, the smell coming out from the mouth of a fasting person is better in the sight of Allah than the smell of musk. [Allah says about the fasting person], 'He has left his food, drink and desires for My sake. The fast is for Me. So I will reward [the fasting person] for it and the reward of good deeds is multiplied ten times' " (Volume 3, Book 31, Number 117).

Fasting for me, a Christian, is also an attempt to sacrifice and commune with the Lord regarding issues dear to my heart. I found the parallelism of the above passages intriguing and supportive of my Christian beliefs. These scriptural passages and my personal observation led to rule 3.

RULE 3: *EAT A MODERATELY PORTIONED MEAL THE NIGHT BEFORE FASTING.*

Getting past 2 p.m. was difficult until I included in my pre-fasting prayer a request for my hunger to be curbed and an appeal to God to assist me in mastering my mind. I was then able to focus on Him and the purposes of my fast and not on the food and fluids I was abstaining from. The thought to ask God to help focus my mind on Him and the purposes of my fast was reinforced through my religious studies. Here are a few examples that inspired further personal reflection, thought, and fortitude.

There is a Hindu belief that the mind is its own worst enemy; it easily launches off into day dreams and fantasies. To master one's mind means to develop a state of serenity and stillness. Through yoga and meditation, one gains enlightenment by focusing and calming one's mind until one can discover and connect with their "Infinite Self." If you have found your Infinite Self, you have infinite knowledge, and through infinite knowledge you can achieve the ultimate goal of a steadfast and personal relationship with God (2:44, 56, 60, 61, 66–68; 3:7; 5:7, 23, 24; 6:5–7, 10, 15; 6:18–36; 12:8–11; 18:49–55).

Buddha taught in the Dhammapada "All we are is the result of what we have thought." Buddha felt that control over one's mind was essential to overcoming ignorance. This construct of Buddhism can also be found in the Eightfold Path. "Right Mindfulness" is the seventh step of the Eightfold Path on one's journey to enlightenment. As I read the Dhammapada and the Eightfold Path, I remembered the passages I had read in the Seventh-day Adventist Church Manual that impressed upon me that health and dietary choices should be made intelligently. To some degree, one could say that making poor choices is ignorance. Intelligence cannot be completely defined as an absence or lesser degree of education. My point can be clarified by addressing personal choices and harmful health behaviors. For example, most people today have heard that smoking tobacco causes an increased risk for lung cancer, emphysema, and death. So, is one who chooses to smoke still ignorant? *Yes!*

Does my answer surprise you? Do you believe that people who harm themselves fully understand the rippling repercussions that waft through society as a result of their behaviors? If they become ill or die as a result of smoking, do they fully understand how the world will be different because they no longer exist and are unable to make contributions to society? I don't think they do. Even the greatest of men are not omnipresent or omniscient. I believe that as we progress down the path of self-mastery, our level of intelligence and awareness becomes less ignorant or rudimentary. We become more cognizant of life and how each plant, animal, or human contributes to the whole in intrinsic ways that are unfathomable to an unenlightened human mind.

Buddha taught that those who seek enlightenment see things for what they are. In other words, they acknowledge that mankind has carnal desires. And after acknowledging senses and desires that hamper one's progression toward enlightenment, one must keep his mind in control, or he will succumb to and become driven by his body's desires. What I believe Buddha is saying is that if you can acknowledge and identify these desires, you can conquer them. As such, you will no longer be held captive by your cravings. I believe that pure intelligence is comprehension of all things, self-mastery, selflessness, and an unwavering devotion to ultimate truth. As my mind mulled over the different religious passages and sacred texts I had read, one from the Doctrine and Covenants came to mind. It reads, "The glory of God is intelligence, or, in other words, light and truth" (D&C 93:36). What is intelligence? For me, intelligence is

1. A perfect understanding of how the positive and negative consequences of your decisions will affect not only yourself and those close to you but also those miles away or years into the future.
2. Recognizing that your stewardships are not limited to yourself, your immediate family, or mankind but also to all that comprises the earth and cosmos.
3. Accountability and a personal desire to rectify behaviors of commission and omission toward even the most nominal component of life.
4. Personal sacrifice for the greater good.
5. Truth, power, and divinity.

RULE 4: *BEGIN YOUR FAST WITH PRAYER AND INCLUDE A PLEA TO HEAVENLY FATHER FOR CONTINUED STRENGTH AND AN EYE (OR STOMACH) SINGLE TO GOD AND THE PURPOSES OF YOUR FAST.*

I began my pre-fasting prayer with a plea for Heavenly Father to help me have a calm and focused mind. My prayer was answered! I was able to successfully fast until 2 p.m. without hunger, headache, or irritability. I was also able to focus my whirlwind of a mind on Heavenly Father and the purpose of my fast instead of food and all of the other activities of daily living that a wife and mother routinely engages in. I can't tell you how satisfied I was on the day that I finally could cook lunch for my non-fasting family members and not absentmindedly taste the food while seasoning it. It was a victory of no small measure for me!

Once I successfully fasted until 2 p.m., the next step was to fast until dinner. Surprisingly, I could fast easily until dinner and didn't even need my morning drink of water. I felt empowered, and to this day I enjoy a greater degree of physical self-mastery.

Before I leave this topic, I would like to emphasize again that you know your body better than anyone, and as such, I encourage you to listen to your body and pace your fasting accordingly. And finally, remember to seek medical and ecclesiastic advice before fasting.

CHAPTER SIX:

WHAT DOES THIS
ALL MEAN?

I remember asking myself three questions after completing my research. Were there common dietary principles among the religions I investigated? What religious dietary principles were supported by science? What was I going to do with this information? Once again I created a table (see pages 52–53) to summarize my findings and clarify my thoughts.

After examining the religious and scientific consensus, I decided that it would be prudent to develop dietary rules that would be tailored to my body's needs. I examined each category of food and assessed the areas of agreement among religions and scientific studies. After personally evaluating the soundness of each precept, I determined the depth of my conviction to adhere to each principle.

MEAT AND EGGS

As I examined the table's dietary guidelines for meat and eggs I found that most of the religious and scientific sources suggested limiting meat and egg consumption or abstinence altogether. I knew that I did not want to try veganism again, but I was open to reducing my meat and egg consumption. After all, in the past, it took several months of eating a vegan diet before I felt like tackling a cow. Looking back, I suspect that I had depleted my body's B-vitamin reserves. It didn't seem natural for me to supplement a

Food/Drink Item	Adventist	Buddhism	Hinduism
Meat	Primarily Vegetarian	Difference of Opinion	Avoid
Eggs	Limit ≤ 3 per wk	Difference of Opinion	Avoid
Legumes & Lentils	Moderate	Yes	Healthful
Fruit	Healthful	Yes	Healthful
Vegetables	Healthful	Yes	Healthful
Whole Grains	Healthful	Yes	Healthful
Dairy	Moderate	Difference of Opinion	Healthful
Nuts	Moderate	Yes	Healthful
Fats	Sparingly	No Mention	Harmful (Fried Foods)
Sugars	Sparingly	Honey only	Moderate
Salt	Sparingly	No Mention	Moderate
Alcohol	Abstain	Abstain	Abstain
Illicit Drugs	Abstain	Abstain	Abstain
Coffee & Tea	Abstain	Yes	Moderate
Caffeinated Beverages	Abstain	Yes	Moderate

Food/Drink Item	Judaism	LDS	Muslims	Science
Meat	Limits on type	Limited: In winter or famine	Limits on type	Limits on portion
Eggs	Healthful	No mention	Healthful	Limits on portion
Legumes &Lentils	Healthful	Healthful	Healthful	Yes
Fruit	Healthful	Healthful	Healthful	Yes
Vegetables	Healthful	Healthful	Healthful	Yes
Whole Grains	Healthful	Healthful	Healthful	Yes
Dairy	Healthful, but not with meat	No mention	Healthful	Limits on portion
Nuts	Healthful	Healthful	Healthful	Limits on portion
Fats	No mention	No mention	No mention	Sparingly
Sugars	Honey only	No mention	Honey	Sparingly
Salt	No mention	No mention	No mention	Sparingly
Alcohol	Moderation	Abstain	Abstain	Sparingly
Illicit Drugs	Abstain	Abstain	Abstain	Abstain
Coffee & Tea	Yes	Abstain	Yes	Sparingly
Caffeinated Beverages	Yes	Abstain	Yes	Sparingly

vegan diet with manufactured B vitamins, so the only other option was to eat meat and eggs and determine the minimum amount my body required for optimal functioning.

I began my experiment by eliminating meats and eggs from my breakfast meal. I did just fine eating grains for breakfast. For lunch and dinner, I ate meat entrées, but after about two weeks, I missed not having an occasional egg for breakfast. So I changed my diet to include an egg for breakfast when I wanted one and then enjoyed a vegetarian lunch and a meat entrée for dinner. It worked well. In fact, I never even missed not having meat at lunch.

Over time, a fascinating physical response developed. My desire for meat has naturally and slowly decreased to where I currently have one egg for breakfast about six to eight times a month in the winter and two to four times a month in the summer. I generally eat a vegetarian breakfast and lunch and enjoy a 5-ounce serving of meat (about the size of a deck of cards or the size of the palm of my hand) for dinner. I like meat nearly every day in the winter and only three to four times a week in the summer. During the winter of 2009, I kept a two-week food diary (see page 86) that may be of benefit if you need ideas for menus; however, please remember that my portion sizes may not be appropriate for your body needs due to differences in our activity levels and body sizes, so use it only as a guide. What you really need to do is become an expert on your own body's specific requirements.

Upon closer examination of my natural appetite for meat and eggs, I discovered that I desired more meat and eggs in the colder months and less meat and eggs in the warmer months. This interesting phenomenon parallels to some degree the teachings found in the Word of Wisdom of the Church of Jesus Christ of Latter-day Saints: "And it is pleasing unto me that [meat] should not be used, only in times of winter, or of cold, or famine."

GRAINS, VEGETABLES, LENTILS, LEGUMES, AND FRUIT

Without fail, every religious sect and scientific study agreed that whole grains, vegetables, lentils, legumes, and fruit were beneficial and should be the bulk of one's diet. Based on my original decision to limit my meat intake to one serving of eggs or 4–5 ounces of meat a day, I needed to figure out what I would be eating in the place of meat. The obvious answer for me was whole grains, lentils, legumes, and vegetables. When I say whole grains, I am not referring to whole wheat bread. What I decided to do was eat pulse (grains and legumes), like Jacob, Daniel, and other biblical characters did; after all, I was taught as a child that God is not a respecter of persons, so if it worked for those in ancient times, why wouldn't it work for me? I attempted to find a biblical recipe for pulse, but I couldn't find one, so I decided to make my own. My recipe consisted of cooked grains, such as whole wheat berries, quinoa, buckwheat, barley, brown rice, lentils, squash, and so on, as well as black beans, kidney beans, northern beans, and garbanzo beans.

I thought it would be wise to increase my vegetable intake as well. My initial plan was to make vegetable side dishes to accompany my pulse entrée. When I tasted my first batch of pulse, I discovered it had a wonderful texture. The grains were firm but soft enough to be comfortably chewed; in fact, they were fun to eat because the wheat berries kind of squeaked as I chewed them. The flavor of each grain was unique, and when eaten together, they resulted in a harmonious blend of nutty but bland flavors. I needed to add some zip or I knew I would never continue my newly developed diet past the initial serving. I wanted to limit my saturated fat intake, so topping my pulse with sauces or dressings was out of the question; instead, I used flavorful raw vegetables and herbs, such as bell peppers, tomatoes, cucumbers, cilantro, basil, rosemary, green onions, garlic, and so forth to spice up my pulse. For a change of pace, I added a bouillon cube to the cooking water and a splash of balsamic vinegar, seasoning sauce, or flavor salt before serving. As a side note, I am especially fond of quinoa. It cooks quickly and is a plant-based complete protein. Lentils also cook quickly.

In addition to my pulse and vegetable–style entrée, I further increased my vegetable intake by adding a side salad or an additional serving of raw, baked, or steamed vegetables. I have never liked butter on my vegetables, so reducing saturated fat was never an issue. I do, however, subscribe to one exception: every summer, my corn on the cob must be slathered in fresh, creamy butter and salt and pepper before I will eat it.

DAIRY

Ascertaining the amount and type of dairy products I would include in my diet was perhaps the most difficult of all because there was not much consensus between religious practice or scientific study. After reading the USDA Food Pyramid recommendations, I decided to decrease the my dairy intake from six to eight cups of milk a day, a cup of yogurt, and an ounce or two of cheese to one cup of milk, a half cup of yogurt, a half cup of cottage cheese, and one ounce of cheese per day.

> **CAUTION:** If any of my readers are dieticians please skip to the next section titled *Sugar and Processed Foods,* as I am certain you are going to go bang your head against the wall if you read further.

I thought I would try incorporating skim milk in my diet, so I bought some and literally spat the "white water" into the kitchen sink! The following week I bought some 2% milk, and it was a little more palatable but not good enough to drink more than a swallow, so I mixed it with whole milk, and it tasted better. Even when I am out of fresh milk, I make my powdered milk stronger than what is called for. I have determined that I am and always will be a whole milk drinker. This is one dietary habit I refuse to modify. Should I have chosen to drink reduced fat milk? Yes! Does the USDA suggest drinking reduced fat milk? Yes! Am I willing to make the switch? NO! Having expressed my deep devotion to whole milk, I think it is now time to move on to the next topic.

But before I do, dieticians, please place this book on your desk, go to the freezer, pull out an ice pack, and place it on your forehead. Next, call the handyman to fix the hole you made in your wall after reading about my devotion to whole milk. After you have completed your call, please continue to read where you left off and remember, I gave you fair warning.

SUGARS AND PROCESSED FOODS

After examining my research findings, I decided to eliminate processed foods and sugars from my diet. I based my decision firmly on the scientific studies discussed in this book as well as biblical examples and my personal belief that God made natural, sweet-tasting foods that are specifically engineered for the health of mankind. For me, this meant that I would not eat sugar but would instead sweeten my morning hot, whole-grain cereals with a small amount of honey or fruit and nuts. I would also abstain from processed foods, candy, pastries, and so forth and instead enjoy a piece of fruit for a snack or dessert.

CAFFEINE, COFFEE, TEA, ALCOHOL, AND DRUGS

Undeniably, religious and scientific studies have demonstrated that caffeinated beverages, strong alcoholic beverages, and illicit drugs are harmful to one's body. I have never had the desire to try illicit drugs and did not like the taste of caffeinated teas, black coffee, or alcoholic drinks. So after I had my fleeting curiosities satisfied, I never desired another sip of these beverages again. However, I do enjoy a certain caffeinated beverage that I affectionately refer to as, "The Nectar of the Gods." If I was going to abstain from processed and sugar-laden foods, I regretfully had to abstain from Coke as well. This was not going to be easy or enjoyable. But I knew if it improved my health and eliminated my chronic constipation, it would be well worth the sacrifice.

CHAPTER SEVEN:

THE W.O.W. DIET
RULES

STOP SEVEN: THE BEST ROUTE TO DIETARY ENLIGHTENMENT IS IN AN INFOMERCIAL?

After being on the my diet for about a month, I had dropped a from a size 14 pant to a size 12. One night, as I was getting ready for bed, Trent stared at me and said that I was "looking fine!" and wanted to know what I was doing differently. I told him in great detail about my research and diet. Trent had the nerve to interrupt my monologue by saying, "Honey, I'm tired. Can't you just give me the nitty-gritty? You know, give me the basic concept and a few rules." Sufficiently annoyed, I informed him that I researched religious dietary words of wisdom as well as empirical evidence supported by dietary research. From that point forward, Trent and I referred to my new diet as the "Words of Wisdom" (W.O.W.) Diet. I further explained to Trent that my W.O.W. Diet plan consisted of ten simple and easy-to-follow rules. When I said this, Trent laughed and said I sounded like an infomercial. So for you readers that want the nitty-gritty of the W.O.W. Diet, here you go!

RULE 1: ENJOY A VARIETY OF WHOLE GRAINS, LENTILS, BEANS, FRESH FRUIT, AND VEGETABLES. THEY ARE INEXPENSIVE, TASTY, FILLING, AND EASY TO PREPARE! THESE SHOULD BE THE BULK OF YOUR MEAL.

***RULE 2: EAT ONLY UNTIL YOU ARE NO LONGER EXPERIENCING
HUNGER PANGS.*** IF YOU ARE UNCERTAIN, WAIT TEN MINUTES
AND SEE IF YOU ARE STILL HUNGRY. BE HONEST WITH YOURSELF!
REMEMBER, DO NOT STARVE YOURSELF; EAT ONLY ENOUGH
FOOD SO THAT IN THREE TO FOUR HOURS YOU ARE READY FOR
A *LIGHT* SNACK.

We have all had friends, coworkers, or loved ones who go on restrictive fad diets. What usually happens? They gain weight over time
and more often than not, they end up weighing more than they
did before they started. This unfortunate phenomenon of post-diet
weight gain has been documented by scientific research involving
men, women, young adults, and children.

Since beginning the W.O.W. Diet, I have never been hungry.
I also unconsciously started eating less food. That is, as long as I
ate whole grain natural foods and listened to my body's hunger and
satiety rhythm, I unconsciously decreased my portion sizes. It has
been three years since I started the W.O.W. Diet, and I have kept my
weight off and continue to lose a few more pounds and inches each
year. In 2010, I was down to a size 9/10 pant.

RULE 3: START YOUR DAY OFF RIGHT . . . EAT BREAKFAST!

Over the years, I noticed that if I skipped breakfast, I ate larger portions and snacked throughout the day. For years, I've heard that
breakfast was the most important meal of the day. I decided to take
some time and research on www.pubmed.gov if there was any empirical research to support this claim. I identified many studies using
the words, "Skipping breakfast and obesity." Over and over again,
research concluded that study participants—adults and children
alike—who skipped breakfast had a greater risk for obesity.

My breakfast consists of hot grain cereals such as steel-cut oats,
fresh ground farina, six grain cereal, quinoa, barley, whole wheat,
teff, brown rice, buckwheat, and fresh ground millet. I sweeten my
cereals with a half cup milk or yogurt and add dried or fresh fruit, a
spoonful of raw nuts, or a teaspoon of honey. I eat an egg about once
a week on the average and whole grain wheat, barley, corn, rye or
multi-grain pancakes once a week. I begin my morning with a warm
mug of water. Sometimes, if I have congestion, I add fresh squeezed

lemon juice. Other times I have some unsweetened peppermint or spearmint tea. Why do I do this? Tradition! My maternal and paternal grandmothers both drank warm water in the morning and as a little girl I joined. My habit is a result of their examples, nothing more. Now that I am a grown woman, I question the benefits of certain behaviors I have adopted over the years.

I researched if temperature of foods or beverages had effect on gastric or bowel motility. I found several older articles that were of questionable merit due to small sample sizes; nonetheless, what was concluded was that food and fluid temperatures made little difference in terms of gastric emptying or motility. I wish I could ask my grandmothers what their rationale was for starting their mornings with a cup of warm water, but I can't. They have both passed on.

RULE 4: EAT AT REGULAR INTERVALS.

I strive to eat my meals at regular times based on what my body desires. I speculated that if my body desired foods more frequently and I ate just to the point of having my hunger pangs eliminated, I would consume fewer calories and lose weight. I researched if increased meal frequency was inversely related to obesity and not surprisingly, it was.

My meal schedule looks like this: breakfast at 6:30 a.m., lunch at 11:00 a.m., a snack at 3 p.m., and dinner at 6 p.m. I also try to sit down at a table for my meals instead of eating on the run or behind the steering wheel of my car. This gives me time to think about my food in terms of Buddha's Five Contemplations of Eating, which we discussed earlier. My husband recently started the W.O.W. Diet and this is his schedule: breakfast at 7 a.m., a light snack such as a hard boiled egg or a 1-ounce cheese stick at 10 a.m., lunch around 12:00 noon, a piece of fruit at 3 p.m., and dinner at 6 p.m.

RULE 5: EAT VEGETARIAN OR LACTO-OVO-VEGETARIAN FOR TWO MEALS A DAY.

Breakfast and lunch range from lacto-ovo-vegetarian to vegetarian meals. If I cannot have a vegetarian lunch out of a desire for meat or an unavailability of vegetarian entrées, I prepare a vegetarian dinner. The recipes at the end of this book include several satisfying and flavorful recipes that I created for my family's enjoyment.

RULE 6: EAT MEAT SPARINGLY.

Dinner may include a combination of vegetables, grains, legumes, beans, potatoes, or fruit but also a small amount of meat, poultry, or fish. I usually eat a 5-ounce (the size of the palm of my hand) serving of meat. When my protein comes in the form of eggs, I usually limit myself to one egg and at times, two. As I mentioned previously, my appetite for meat and eggs has decreased over the last few months and changes with the seasons.

RULE 7: EAT FOODS IN THEIR NATURAL STATE WHENEVER POSSIBLE.

I allow myself as many servings of fresh, raw, steamed, baked, or stir-fried vegetables as I want. I generally eat about a half cup to one cup of green salad, a half cup of vegetables, and three-fourths to one cup combined whole grains, squash, legumes, and/or beans. I tend to eat two pieces of fruit a day; usually one for my 3 p.m. snack and another serving at dinner. I also eat dairy in the form of cultured milk, such as a half cup yogurt or buttermilk, half cup cottage cheese, or one ounce hard cheese. When I want it, I drink a cup of pasteurized milk. Though I eat an assortment of dairy products, the majority of my dairy servings are from homemade yogurt to which I add probiotics (helpful bacteria). I decided to switch from most of my dairy coming from pasteurized whole milk to eating yogurt supplemented with probiotics after reading three randomized control trials that reported decreased constipation in study participants receiving cultured milk and/or probiotic supplements.

As a side note, if you choose to read the probiotics studies referenced in the bibliography, do not become alarmed, as a friend of mine did, after reading that the scientists administered Escherichia Coli (E. Coli) bacteria to study participants. There are many strains of E. Coli; most are not harmful to humans, and as is the case of probiotics, some may be beneficial. However, other strains of E. Coli are harmful when ingested by humans, such as E. Coli strain 0157 or E. Coli serotypes 026, 0111, and 0103. When ingested, these strains can cause symptoms ranging from abdominal cramps, diarrhea, and low-grade fever to kidney failure and death. For more information on E. Coli and how to better protect yourself from harmful strains of E. Coli, please visit the Centers for Disease Control and Prevention (CDC) website at www.cdc.gov/ecoli/.

RULE 8: IT'S OKAY TO HAVE A LIGHT AND HEALTHFUL SNACK ONCE OR TWICE A DAY IN BETWEEN MEALS.

I believe that I am programmed for a snack in the afternoon because some days, I am not even hungry, but I have a desire to eat something.

During my childhood years, my dear mother would always have a delicious and often sweet snack on the kitchen bar for me to eat when I returned home from school at precisely 3 p.m. I have great memories of my mother sitting down on a kitchen stool beside me and asking about my day. It was a wonderful time for me to refuel and visit with Mom before running off to play. Now I am an adult woman who still needs to snack at 3! In the past, I tried to fight the urge to have something to eat, but eventually I wisened up and acknowledged that for whatever reason, I needed an afternoon snack.

Once I came to this pragmatic point of view, I stopped fighting my body and began working with it instead. A snack every day was fine, but choice of food needed to change. The W.O.W. Diet no longer allowed me to reach for sweet treats such as cookies, brownies, or a bowl of ice cream. My snacks now consist of healthier food choices such as a slice of cheese, six to eight nuts, a half cup yogurt, a piece of fruit, vegetables, a cup of salad, or, on rare occasions, a 4-ounce smoothie made of homemade yogurt and fruit.

RULE 9: MAKE WATER YOUR BEVERAGE OF CHOICE AND CONSUME IT LIBERALLY!

Water quenches thirst, has no calories, and cleanses and replenishes our bodies. I drink six to eight glasses of water throughout the day in the winter and eight to ten glasses of water in the summer. Water is my beverage of choice, and I hope it will soon become yours as well.

RULE 10: AVOID REFINED CARBOHYDRATES, CONCENTRATED SUGARS, AND FAT-FRIED OR PROCESSED FOODS!

As I mentioned earlier, I rarely eat foods that have been refined or processed by man like prepared breakfast cereals, white flour breads, pastas, muffins, cookies, brownies, pies, cakes, ice cream, candy, soft drinks, and so forth. This wasn't easy because I loved having dessert after each evening meal. Once I decided to abstain from these foods, I quickly discovered that refined foods are everywhere and are frequently the only food choices available at social gatherings. I remember breathing in the wonderful aroma of fresh baked pastries, cakes, and cookies. It was difficult because I did not require my family to join me on this dietary adventure, and they would freely indulge in treats in front of me.

Do I ever eat fast food or have an occasional potato chip or other treat? Absolutely! Who doesn't? Once a week, my family orders takeout, brings home pizza, or goes out for burgers. When we order takeout, it's usually Asian cuisine. When we order pizza, I typically eat one slice of pizza and about a cup of green salad. When we go for burgers, I order a junior hamburger, without cheese or bacon, eat six or eight fries, and drink lots of water.

Occasionally, we enjoy a nice, sit-down dinner at a restaurant. I will pay for an additional side salad and divide my entrée with Trent, or we both order and take home leftovers.

SUMMARY OF THE W.O.W. DIET RULES

Rule 1	Make the bulk of your diet grains, lentils, beans, vegetables, and fruit.
Rule 2	Eat only enough to satisfy hunger.
Rule 3	Eat breakfast.
Rule 4	Eat at regular intervals.
Rule 5	Make two of three meals vegetarian or if necessary lacto-ovo-vegetarian.
Rule 6	Eat small portions of meat.
Rule 7	Eat foods in their natural state when possible.
Rule 8	Allow yourself to eating small, healthy snacks between meals.
Rule 9	Make water your beverage of choice.
Rule 10	Avoid refined carbohydrates, concentrated sugars, and fat-fried or processed foods.

HELPFUL TIDBITS

CHANGE YOUR DEFINITION OF FAST FOOD

In the past, I've challenged my husband to drive to a fast food restaurant two miles from our home, order a meal, and make it back home in the same amount of time it would take me to make a nutritious, home-cooked meal. In twenty minutes, Trent had his dinner in a bag on the dinning room table. I too had my dinner ready in twenty minutes without leaving the comfort of my home or spending money on gas.

Trent's dinner consisted of two small cheeseburgers with bacon, an order of fries, and a soft drink. My dinner included a tilapia filet, a microwaved potato, a green salad, and some orange slices. Trent ate his dinner, said he was still hungry, and asked if I would share. Not only did I serve Trent some of my tilapia, but I also dished him up a very smug grin.

I believe that eating healthy is more often than not a matter of choice and organization rather than convenience. When you first begin the W.O.W. Diet, you may have difficulties finding time to cook whole grains, or perhaps you have never made homemade yogurt. Here are a few simple and time efficient tips to get you started along your path of dietary enlightenment.

- Once a month, I purchase a month's worth of the following root and squash vegetables: carrots, parsnips, turnips, beets, yellow onions, garlic, potatoes, jicama, cabbage, spaghetti squash, acorn squash, and butternut squash.

- Once a week, I buy vegetables with a shorter shelf life: cilantro, basil, oregano, lettuce, spinach, tomatoes, cucumbers, green onions, broccoli, cauliflower, bell peppers, avocado, zucchini, and yellow squash.

- Once a week, I buy bananas, citrus, apples, and, *if in season and reasonably priced,* fresh grapes, kiwis, melons, pineapple, peaches, pears, plums, apricots, strawberries, raspberries, blueberries, and blackberries. During the winter, I buy frozen berries.

As a result of my shopping routine, I have greater inventory control. I only buy what our family will eat over the shelf life of the produce (which eliminates waste) and am able to provide plenty of wholesome fresh fruits and vegetables for my family to enjoy.

There is one oddity that I can't seem to grasp. If I buy four bananas, my family of four will eat the bananas in two days and ask for more. As a result of their gobbling up the bananas in two days, the next time I go to the grocery store I buy eight bananas. If you have experienced this same situation, you know what happens. My family will eat all but two bananas, so the following week, I cut back to six bananas. And to no surprise, they complain that I didn't buy enough bananas and could I please buy more next time. So I buy seven bananas. By the end of the week, I have two brown, soft bananas sitting in the fruit bowl.

I have talked to my girlfriends about this banana conundrum, and they too have difficulties figuring out how many bananas to buy for their families. So you know what I do? I buy six bananas each week. When they are gone, I say, "Tough luck, eat something else." Situation remedied!

Another convenient and money-saving tip is to buy grains, lentils and beans in twenty-five to fifty-pound bags. Or, buy your grains and lentils in bulk bags and canned beans during case lot sales.

Price check bulk items at grocery stores and health food stores before you make your purchase. You will be surprised at how much food prices vary. Many stores will order bulk twenty-five to fifty-pound sacks of grains, lentils, or beans for you even if they don't have a bulk section in their store.

Ask for a 10-percent discount when buying large quantities. Remember to negotiate the discount before you commit to buying. I usually say something like this. "I see your salmon is on sale for $3.99 a pound. If I buy 50 pounds, may I have 10 percent off the price?" Or "Could you tell me what the price per pound is for a 25-pound bag of red lentils, yellow lentils, green lentils, barley pearls, wheat berries, and quinoa? If I buy all of this today, may I have 10-percent off the price?"

Always prepay for your order in full. Food prices are escalating at such a fast pace that the price of your order may go up several dollars before it arrives at the store. If you prepay for your order, the store will honor the quoted price, regardless of any increases.

Cook your grains, beans, rice, lentils, and squash once or twice a week and then store them in the refrigerator for future use. I spend an hour and a half cooking my grains and squash for the week. I start with the squash because it takes forty-five minutes to one hour to cook in the oven. Once the squash has been placed in the oven, I turn to the grains that have the longest cooking time. Wheat berries take about an hour to an hour and half to cook on the stove top. Once I get them cooking, I set the oven timer for an hour and a half. Next I get my barley pearls simmering; they take an hour to cook. When the barley pearls are simmering, I set the timer on the microwave for an hour. Next I cook brown rice in the rice cooker. While everything is simmering, I soak and rinse the quinoa. When the brown rice is finished cooking, I place it in a bowl, clean out the rice cooker, and start the quinoa in the rice cooker. Lentils are the last item that I prepare because they only require ten minutes to cook on the stove top.

After all of my grains are cooked, I place them in sealed containers in the refrigerator. I also chop assorted raw flavorful vegetables to be used as toppers or garnishes such as cilantro, basil, green onions, tomatoes, peppers, and so forth.

During the week, if I want grains for breakfast, I simply spoon out what I want, reheat, and enjoy. If I need grains or lentils for lunch, in an entrée, or as a snack, I merely spoon out what I need, and in a matter of seconds I have a delicious meal.

As far as beans go, I do not cook dried beans because I do not like the smell. I buy my beans in cans. For the sake of convenience, I open the cans of beans I want to eat for the week while my grains are cooking, rinse them thoroughly, and place the beans in air tight containers in the refrigerator.

I make homemade yogurt twice a month without a yogurt machine. It takes about thirty minutes to prepare and three to four hours to ripen in the oven, so if I am pressed for time, I make my yogurt before going to bed. Once the liquid yogurt is made, I place the containers in an oven with the light on and close the door. In the morning, I wake up, take the ripened yogurt out of the oven, place it in the refrigerator, and head off to work. My total cost per gallon of yogurt is the cost of a gallon of milk ($1.85–$2.50).

Once you've added delicious and nutritious fresh fruit and vegetables, your meal of whole grains, lentils, beans, and yogurt is fast and easy if purchased and made in advance.

EXERCISE

I have been asked on numerous occasions if I have an established exercise routine. My answer is, "Kind of." I don't like to exercise. However, I do like to play, and I like to complete purposeful activities. What that means is I exercise best when it is fun and when I can accomplish more things than just working out. For example, I wanted to save money and get some exercise. After giving my desires some thought, I bought Sebastian. Sebastian is an amazing adult tricycle that has a large basket on the back. Sebastian's basket holds a week's worth of groceries for our family of four, plus dry cleaning, mail, items from the hardware store, and so on.

When the weather is nice, I ride Sebastian around town, completing my errands. My rides are only about four to six miles, round trip, but I feel refreshed and energized by the time I return home. I do not ride in high winds, when it is raining, or once the winter snow has arrived. I plan my errands anytime between 9 a.m. and 2 p.m. because I do not enjoy riding a bike the size of a banana boat in heavier traffic.

It's fun riding Sebastian because I have made many friends as I peddle around town completing my errands. Other bikers, riding their expensive touring bikes and wearing spandex, wave and give me the "hang loose" sign. Shopkeepers and customers smile and wave. Life is good when I am out and about with Sebastian; I hear the birds singing, I feel the sunshine and a gentle breeze on my face, and more importantly, I feel more connected with my environment and community. I never realized what simple pleasures I was missing out on as I drove around town inside my air-conditioned car listening to my favorite CD.

In addition to peddling Sebastian around town several days a week, I use free weights one to two times a week in an attempt to maintain my upper body strength. I also practice yoga two to three days a week. During the summer, we take our dog Izzie on walks, hike, and play at the lake and mountains. In the winter, we occasionally go bowling, take Izzie on short walks, go dancing a couple times a month, and snow ski. Exercise for me is not a routine that I grudgingly do. Exercise for me must be a part of my daily activities, and above all, it must be enjoyable!

CHAPTER EIGHT:

PERSONAL
OUTCOMES

STOP 8: HAVE I ARRIVED?

I would never have considered myself as being addicted to anything; however, after what I experienced over the first three weeks of the W.O.W. Diet, I can now tell you that I was addicted to Coke, chocolate in any form, brownies, ice cream, and pastries. In other words, I was addicted to processed carbohydrates and simple sugars. I had cravings while I was awake that were so strong that it took all I had not to grab a treat from a passing toddler and devour it like a wild beast. When I attended social gatherings, I could smell the dessert buffet with such clarity that I would begin salivating as I told Trent each item I could smell. I even had dreams about eating my forbidden foods.

I queried "carbohydrates and sugar addiction" in a web search. Unfortunately, at this point in time, scientists do not have enough empirical evidence to classify humans demonstrating addictive food behaviors such as binging, craving, and withdrawals under the category of substance dependence. However, research scientists using animal modeling, case control studies, neurochemistry, and observational data are finding evidence that suggests processed foods containing high amounts of sugar, sweeteners, refined carbohydrates, salt, and fats may become addictive to certain individuals.

Giving up refined and sugary foods was difficult beyond my

wildest imagination, but somewhere around the end of week three, my cravings ended. I was no longer tempted, much to the chagrin of my children who loved taunting me with some Baskin Robbins chocolate peanut butter ice cream or homemade chocolate chocolate chip brownies. I truly know that what kept me from caving to my cravings were the positive outcomes I began experiencing a few days into the W.O.W. Diet.

Almost immediately, I started passing gas throughout the day. Three days into the W.O.W. Diet, I passed a small, hard-formed bowel movement without the use of laxatives. After a week, I was defecating fluffy, easily passed stools one or two times a day. I began feeling really good. I was no longer experiencing abdominal pains in the lower right quadrant of my abdomen. My abdominal girth was decreasing. I had more energy. I was sleeping better at night, and I had an increased desire for sexual intimacy with my husband. I was feeling healthy, vibrant, and alive, and that feeling is what empowered me to stay away from my forbidden foods. Not only did I receive these health benefits from the W.O.W. Diet but I also received secondary benefits as well.

THEY MAY LOOK DAZZLING BUT ONE WHIFF AND YOU ARE A GONER!

Every morning when the alarm clock rings, I cuddle up to my husband's back for fifteen minutes, get out of bed, brush my teeth, kiss my husband, and wake the children. Why do I brush my teeth before I kiss my husband good morning? Because every morning without fail, I have a thick layer of plaque on my teeth and the most killer dragon breath imaginable. You may be thinking, *Lady, have you ever tried flossing and brushing your tongue and teeth before you go to bed?*

I have meticulous oral hygiene, but my breath has made my children gag and my husband ask me to gargle. That is until one morning about a month after beginning the W.O.W. Diet, I noticed that I hadn't brushed my teeth and had kissed Trent and the children good morning with no untoward effects.

The next morning, I began experimenting and researching scientific articles on dental hygiene. I placed my hand to my mouth and breathed, but I couldn't detect any foul odors. I ran my tongue across my teeth, and they felt as though I had just brushed them. I had Trent sniff my breath. Much to his reluctance, he sniffed and was surprised when my breath smelled fresh. What had changed? My diet.

As I examined the changes in my mouth and teeth, I realized that what I had done was eliminate, for the greater part, processed carbohydrates and simple sugars. I had returned to eating foods in their whole or natural state. I wondered if the elimination of the processed carbohydrates and simple sugars decreased the fuel for the natural bacterial flora found in my mouth, namely sticky, sugar-laden foods for bacteria to feed on. I also wondered if my new diet was responsible for the decreased plaque formation and halitosis.

I needed to know more about Westernization of diets and the global impact of dental disease. Please keep in mind that it is perfectly natural for me to make an inquiring leap from a decrease in personal plaque and halitosis to researching globalization of dental disease. If you must roll your eyes, it's okay; my children do it all the time. They also fear that when I gaze at them and write something down on a piece of paper, they have been unknowingly enrolled in a rogue research study by their mother. I just give them a fiendish smile and a sinister laugh and call it payback for their mocking as I secretly write "tomatoes" on my grocery list.

Most Americans know, thanks to the American Dental Association, the US Department of Agriculture, and the American Dietetic Association's educational campaigning, that soft drinks, processed carbohydrates, and sugars not only contribute to the development of a myriad of diseases but also significantly increase the risk of cavities. I was not interested in conducting a basic literature search on diet and tooth decay. I was interested in locating longitudinal studies that incorporated three necessary elements: participants must be young, have lived in a country in which the typical diet consisted of few processed foods and sugar, and the second necessary element was that the scientists must assess dental disease immediately upon arrival to the United States and then again a year or so later. Essentially, I wanted to know if there were any studies examining the relationship between the degree of "Westernization" on a population's diet and an increased rate of tooth decay.

Unfortunately, I was unable to locate such a study. However, three studies were of profound interest. These studies demonstrated support for the argument that "Westernization" of traditional ethnic diets contribute to an increase in tooth decay. MacGregor examined 974 mouths for dental disease. He observed that diets and tooth decay had a direct correlation to socioeconomic status and economic prosperity of towns and villages in Ghana. He identified that study participants living in remote villages experienced a poor standard of living with 22 percent of residents experiencing some form of tooth decay; study participants with a fair standard of living had 44 percent tooth decay, and lastly, 60 percent of those living in more urbanized or acculturated areas and experiencing a good standard of living had some form of tooth decay. In addition, MacGregor found that the consumption of sweets not only doubled the rate of tooth decay—48 percent in sweet eaters as compared to 24 percent in non-sweet eaters—but also increased the severity of tooth decay.

The second study published in 1992 examined Ethiopian refugees' oral health and noted that Ethiopian homeland diets consisted of little or no processed foods or sugar. In addition, Sgan-Cohen et al. reported that none of the refugees had ever seen a dentist before. Still, 86.8 percent of five-year-olds, 81.8 percent of twelve-year-olds and 54 percent of adults were cavity free upon examination!

The last study examined the oral health of refugees from Africa and Eastern Europe. In addition to noting rates of decay, scientists also compared the prevalence of refugee's tooth decay to that of American children. Though there were many studies that examined the prevalence of tooth decay and dental disease among refugees, I was drawn to this study because it demonstrated marked differences in the prevalence of dental decay among refugees from countries with culturally differing diets.

Nearly 225 children between the ages of six months to eighteen years were examined for dental disease. Based on the data collected from the Third National Health and Nutrition Examination Survey (NHANES III) Cote et al. concluded that 38 percent of African refugees, 79.7 percent of Eastern European refugees, and 49.3 percent of US children experienced tooth decay. Furthermore, 62 percent of the African children did not have any sign of tooth decay and were also the least likely to have ever seen a dentist (12.8 percent) or to have owned a toothbrush (10.2 percent). I wonder what the response would have been if researchers would have asked the African children if they had a chewing stick or siwak for dental hygiene. Chewing sticks are effective tools for oral hygiene and are commonly used in Africa, Asia, and the Middle East.

Not surprisingly, only 20.3 percent of Eastern European children were free from dental decay, and 53.8 percent of those received dental care in their home country, and 64.3 percent of them reported that they owned a toothbrush. And lastly, among US children, 50.7 percent did not have tooth decay with no report of the number of US children who have seen a dentist or owned a toothbrush.

I would like to say that diet is the reason for the differences, especially after observing the changes in my own mouth, but one should always consider other slices of the "causal pie," such as genetics, natural occurring fluoride levels in drinking water, oral flora, salivary flow, and cultural practices such as rinsing after eating.

I also performed a literature search on the association between halitosis and processed foods and sugar consumption in diets but came up empty-handed. Most of the twenty-four research articles addressed odor-producing bacteria and foods that cause malodorous breath such as milk, garlic, and onions—all of which I have continued to enjoy.

Lastly, I researched vegetarian diets and dental decay. One study examined the relationship between tooth decay and parental literacy and income, vegetarian and non-vegetarian diets, oral hygiene methods, and sweet consumption. In summary, Venugopal et al. found that children who were eating a vegetarian diet, who limited consumption of sweets, and who rinsed their mouths after eating had the lowest prevalence of tooth decay. They also noted that children who used a chewing stick had the least amount of tooth decay when compared to those who used a toothbrush and tooth paste.

Oh, by the way, the last time I had my teeth cleaned, the hygienist said, "You have very little tartar on your teeth. You're doing a great job!" I wanted to respond, "Yes, I am working hard at eating right, and the benefits are amazing."

THE EYES HAVE IT!

Ever since I can remember, I have had people comment on the color of my eyes. My eyes are hazel with yellow lines that extend through my irises into billowing rings around the inner and outer edges. One morning, approximately three months after beginning the W.O.W. Diet, I was putting on mascara and noticed that my eye coloring had changed. No longer did I have prominent yellow lines extending through my irises. In addition to this oddity, the billowing yellow rings had faded and were smaller. At first I thought my eye changes were created by the color of my eye shadow or the blouse I was wearing.

As I pondered the visible changes in my eyes, a very old memory came to mind. My first marriage occurred in 1984. My husband and I were given an unusual wedding gift by one of my husband's sisters. Her gift to us was an eye reading. I thanked her for the gift and in a scoffing manner told my husband that he needed to keep an open mind. If nothing else, we might get some entertainment value out of our appointment. About four to five months later, I was scrapbooking our wedding cards, found the eye reading gift certificate, and decided to make an appointment. It turned out to be interesting to say the least. From memory, here is how things transpired.

The woman, I'll call her Susan, told us that she was an iridologist. She said iridology was the study of the iris. Through examining a person's iris, she would be able to identify systems within our bodies that were strong or weak.

Next, we were seated in upright chairs and told to relax as Susan shined a light into each eye and spoke about what she was seeing. Susan told me that my irises had a great deal of yellow in them and that this was a manifestation of a malfunctioning and unhealthy gastrointestinal tract. I remember being surprised at hearing this. I quickly chalked it up to my visibly distended abdomen. However, what came out of her mouth next was shocking. Susan told me that I *had* had a traumatic birth and was resuscitated. My mouth literally fell open at hearing this! I *did* have a traumatic birth! Both my mother and I had to be resuscitated. I asked her how she knew, and she told me that my iris revealed that I had been without oxygen at birth. Each of our appointments lasted an hour and a half. During this time, many other health issues were suggested. Several of the diagnoses were accurate.

On the ride home, my husband and I were both mystified by the accuracy of the past and present body strengths, illnesses, and areas of concern she had identified. It was an intriguing experience, and we both wondered if Susan was a psychic or if she delved into the paranormal. After a few weeks, however, I forgot about this experience until 2007, when my eye coloring began to change.

My curiosity about iridology was rekindled, which lead to yet another literature search. I was surprised to find thirty-five iridology research articles. Thirteen of these articles were in foreign languages. Of the remaining twenty-two research articles, eleven of them were accessible through our local university library. Two of the eleven research articles were review articles examining iridology and its validity as a diagnostic tool. I assessed each of the nine remaining research articles for soundness of study design, appropriateness of methodology, and validity of conclusions. After evaluating each article for scholarly merit, three of the eleven published research articles, though limited by important methodological issues, could be considered scientific studies.

Allie Simon et al. (1979) designed a case control study in which ninety-five of the participants were free of kidney disease (controls) and forty-eight had kidney disease (cases). To begin, 35 mm slides were taken of the participants' eyes. Three iridologists and three ophthalmologists viewed the slides and were asked to determine which participants had kidney disease. After the diagnostic responses were analyzed, both the iridologists and ophthalmologists demonstrated a statistically insignificant ability to diagnose kidney disease in participants.

In 1988, the British Medical Journal published a study by Paul Knipschild that tested the ability of iridologists to diagnose gall bladder disease. Thirty-nine study participants had confirmed gall bladder disease (cases) and thirty-nine participants were free from gall bladder disease (controls). Confirmation of disease was confirmed through ultrasound imaging. Slides were taken of each participant's right eye and shown to five iridologists. Once again, as demonstrated by Simon's earlier kidney disease study, iridologist's diagnostic abilities were nearly equal to that of chance.

The last study researched the ability of iridologists to diagnose cancer. Sixty-eight study participants had laboratory confirmed cancers (cases). Forty-two study participants were cancer free (controls). Of the participants with a laboratory-confirmed cancer, the iridologist only identified three correctly. It would have been interesting for the researchers to conduct a prospective study to determine if those participants who were cancer free at the time of the study later developed cancer in the organs identified by the iridologist. Nonetheless, three correctly diagnosed cancer participants out of a total of sixty-eight is not a significant argument for iridology as a diagnostic tool.

After reading the above published research articles, I was, and still remain, puzzled by the changes of my eye coloring and the diagnostic abilities of Susan. Why were my irises no longer streaked with yellow? Did the W.O.W. Diet really cause the color change, or was it just coincidence? What was different about Susan's skill, knowledge, and diagnostic abilities? And lastly, what would Susan's diagnostic accuracy have been if she would have participated in the kidney, gall bladder, and cancer studies?

After being faithful to the W.O.W. Diet for a year, my weight decreased from 186 pounds to 154 pounds. The other day, my husband asked if I was ever hungry since being on the W.O.W. Diet. My answer was no. I have not felt hungry; in fact, I have greater satiety, which is the feeling of fullness between meals. I asked Trent why he was asking me if I was hungry, and he said that he noticed that I eat smaller portions of food. I was unaware that I had decreased my food portions over time, but when I thought about it, I had.

When I first began the W.O.W. Diet, I would reach for a seven-inch bowl and heap it up with food. Now I eat from a five-inch bowl and rarely fill it to the top. I wish I could remember when I transitioned serving sizes, but I can't. What I can tell you is this: *I will not suffer from hunger if I have anything to do with it!* The exception to this is when I choose to fast for religious purposes. What does all of this mean? It means that for me to decrease my serving size, it had to have been a natural and unconscious behavior that did not include the unpleasant consequence of hunger pangs.

It is interesting to note that before beginning the W.O.W. Diet, I often wasn't satisfied after eating a meal. I sometimes went to the kitchen, opened the pantry and refrigerator, and stared into them for a while. I said to my family, "I'm hungry for something, but I just can't figure out what it is." They would make suggestions, but nothing they suggested would satisfy my desire for food. Interestingly, I have rarely finished a meal and felt hungry for something else since beginning the W.O.W. Diet.

In an attempt to find answers to this phenomenon I conducted a literature search by entering "Dietary fiber and satiety." One hundred seventy-three scholarly articles appeared. Needless to say, there is a plethora of research examining and demonstrating that fiber increases satiety, but the question remained: why was I still hungry for some unknown something before the W.O.W. Diet? I ate high-fiber foods, drank fiber supplements, and even took fiber pills.

My next thought was to research carbohydrates and their ranking on the glycemic index. The glycemic index ranks carbohydrate foods in terms of their ability to raise blood glucose levels within two hours of consumption. Simply stated, low glycemic index foods tend to be carbohydrate foods that are eaten in their natural whole states, whereas high glycemic index foods are refined or processed carbohydrates. Upon entering "Glycemic Index and Satiety," I found eighty-three articles. Many of the articles concluded that low glycemic index foods improved satiety, and a few others cast doubt that low glycemic foods made any difference.

So what could be creating the difference in my satiety and food portion size before and after the W.O.W. Diet? As I reflected on the research I had read and thought about the foods in the W.O.W. Diet, I determined that the W.O.W. Diet consists of high-fiber whole grains, beans, legumes, fresh fruits, and vegetables. We know that high-fiber foods are naturally higher in micronutrients. Micronutrients are vitamins and minerals. Personally, I categorize phytochemicals and enzymes as micronutrients as well; however, phytochemicals and enzymes have not been scientifically proven to be a necessary component of human nutrition and therefore are not "officially" categorized as micronutrients.

Next, I pondered the mechanical process of refining foods. We know that because mechanical processing uses chemicals and high temperatures, many vitamins, minerals, enzymes, and phytochemicals in foods are destroyed. Many food manufacturers—and the US government through the enforcement of regulations—attempt to compensate for the reduction of micronutrients in processed foods by requiring that foods be fortified with micronutrients before packaging. This chain of thoughts led me to contemplate if the actual triggers of satiety are in fact micronutrients. I further questioned whether micronutrients are being confounded due to their natural association with high fiber foods.

This is purely entertaining speculation on my part, but I am willing to hypothesize that the reason for my increased satiety, unconsciously decreasing my serving sizes, and no longer longing for something to eat after a meal is that my body is getting all of the necessary micronutrients it needs. I further hypothesize that if the body is not getting what it needs in terms of micronutrients, it will desire more food in an attempt to obtain them. In other words, the body is hard wired for satiation with a micronutrient closed-loop feedback system.

Notice I did not include the macronutrients fat, fiber, or protein. I didn't include those items because before the W.O.W. Diet, I ate double if not triple the amount of animal fats and proteins that I do now. I also ate copious amounts of high fiber foods and fiber supplements on a daily basis in an attempt to have a bowel movement and still remained hungry. My micronutrient hypothesis could explain why I did not have satiety even though I was on high fiber supplements. Why? Because high fiber supplements do not contain all of the naturally occurring micronutrients available in natural unrefined foods such as whole grains, beans, legumes, fruits, and vegetables.

If we take my micronutrient hypothesis one step further, it may explain why the fast food generation in the United States, which is obese due to eating large amounts of refined carbohydrates and sugar-laden foods, snacks more and eats larger portions. Perhaps this generation is driven into eating more and more food than necessary in an attempt to fill their body's micronutrient needs. In my excitement, I shared my hypothesis with Trent. He thinks in pictures, and so I quickly developed the diagram on the following page.

For those of you who process word explanations better, I am hypothesizing that there are micronutrient (which in my model includes vitamins, minerals, photochemicals, and enzymes) receptors inside the stomach. When a meal is eaten, micronutrients fill the receptors to one degree or another.

If a sufficient amount of micronutrients were in the foods eaten, then the stomach produces a sufficient amount of peptides. In response to these peptides, the pancreas produces a sufficient amount of satiety hormones, which make their way to the brain and create five to six hours of satiation. When the satiety hormones dwindle, the brain sends signals that it is time to eat again. If the opposite is true, if the meal is limited on micronutrients, the stomach's micronutrient receptors do not create enough peptides, and the pancreas responds by producing a limited amount of satiety hormones. A limited amount of pancreatic satiety hormones signals the individual's brain that more food needs to be eaten, and the individual experiences brief satiation of appetite, regardless of the size of the previously ingested meal.

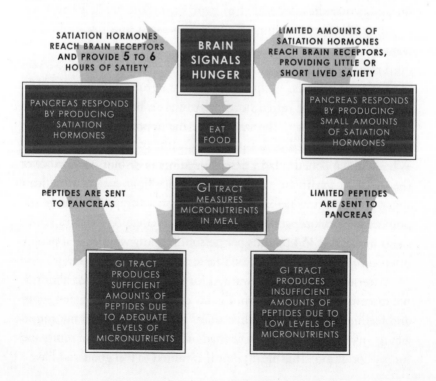

I must reemphasize to my readers that I am not a biomedical scientist; my hypothesis is simply speculation at this point in time. Out of curiosity, I searched pubmed.gov to see if there were any studies addressing micronutrients' effect on satiation of appetite. Unfortunately, I found no empirical research focusing on micronutrients and satiety.

To summarize, nothing I could find within the realm of published scientific literature definitively explained why I had reduced my serving size, experienced greater satiety, and was no longer constipated after committing to the W.O.W. Diet. However, I did have an enjoyable time researching and hypothesizing. And who knows, maybe some day a biomedical research scientist may discover a relationship between micronutrients and satiety, and my future grandchildren will say, "Hey, Grandma was right!"

Even though I could not explain through experimental knowledge why I was no longer chronically constipated, had lost a significant amount of weight, and now felt more vibrant, I truly believe that through the W.O.W. Diet, I found a cure for my gastric and intestinal maladies. I decided to experiment and see if I had been cured. I did this by eating all of the processed and sugary foods I wanted.

I remember the first time I ate a brownie after my year of abstaining from junk foods. I expected pleasure beyond imagination, but instead the brownie tasted horrible! It was sickeningly sweet to the point of tasting bitter. The same thing happened when I took a bite of a candy bar, tried a scoop of ice cream, or took a sip of soda. What had happened? Had I desensitized my taste buds to sugar over the years? According to the Weston A. Price Foundation, American sugar consumption before industrialization was approximately ten pounds per person per year. In 1997, the average American's yearly sugar intake was 154 pounds per person. Is it any wonder that people often complain that fruit doesn't taste as sweet as it used to?

After eating whatever I wanted for a day, I experienced abdominal discomfort and distention. By day three, I was constipated again and feeling horrible. It was then that I realized that I had not found a cure; instead, the W.O.W. Diet had only created a state of remission for my condition. This meant that if I wanted to feel good and have a healthy digestive tract, I would need to make a cultural dietary shift and stay on the W.O.W. Diet for the rest of my life.

Going back on the W.O.W. Diet was difficult as I discovered that my body was once again craving sugary processed foods. I tried to incrementally wean myself off of processed foods and sugar but to no avail. I finally went "cold turkey" and experienced success. Currently, I am abstaining from and no longer crave processed foods or sugars.

I continue to experience the benefits of the enlightening W.O.W. Diet. My health has significantly improved. In 2005, my cholesterol was 235. Three months after being on the W.O.W. Diet my cholesterol dropped to 183 with an HDL (good cholesterol) of 73. I am wearing a size 9/10, down from a tight-fitting size 14 pant (Jan. 2007). When I began the W.O.W. Diet, I weighed 186; presently I weigh 148, a remarkable thirty-eight pound loss.

So far, after being on the W.O.W. Diet for twelve weeks, Trent has lost fourteen pounds and five inches from his waist. My mother, who is seventy two years old and who has suffered with IBS of the diarrheal variety for most of her life, has been on the W.O.W. Diet for three weeks. She has lost twelve pounds and four inches from her waist. And more importantly, she has not had any bouts of diarrhea since beginning the W.O.W. Diet. My stepfather, age 71, is not as faithful to the W.O.W. Diet as my mother, and he's still lost seven pounds in three weeks.

We are all grateful for my husband's wise advice to pray to God for answers; for it was through prayer that my journey led me to dietary words of wisdom given of God and supported by science. I wish I could say that through rigorous clinical trials I discovered a cure for gastrointestinal aliments; but my experience may only be classified as a non-scientific case study at best. However, what I can confidently say about the W.O.W. Diet is that it is a sustainable and sensible approach to a healthier lifestyle through the gentle practice of temperance and better nutrition. In closing, I wish you prosperity, peace, joy, and of course, healthful eating!

CONCLUSION:

W.O.W. YOUR FAMILY

After being on the W.O.W. Diet for a year, I decided to keep a food and exercise diary for two weeks. This was an interesting activity because I don't normally measure my food portions. What immediately struck me after examining my food diary was the proportion of food I eat during a meal in comparison to the size of my stomach. In nursing school, I was taught that an adult stomach can hold between four to six cups of food and fluids.

Notice that I eat an average of about 1½–2 cups of food at any given meal and drink about 2 cups of fluids. This means I'm leaving about 1½–2 cups of my stomach to air as the dietary words of wisdom recorded by the Muslim scholar Muhammad al-Bukhari suggests. Perhaps you remember reading the following passage in my fasting section? ". . . If he has to fill his stomach, then let him leave one-third for food, one-third for drink and one-third for air." (Saheeh al-Jaami' Verse 5,674). Simply by happenstance, I observed a parallel between ancient words of wisdom on food portions and my eating habits after being on the W.O.W. Diet for a year. Fascinating to say the least!

MICHELLE'S W.O.W. DIET DIARY

WEEK ONE:

MONDAY

BREAKFAST: ¾ cup 6-Grain Cereal with ½ teaspoon honey and ½ cup milk.

LUNCH: 1 cup Parsnip Soup and 1 Bran Muffin

SNACK: 1 apple

DINNER: ¾ cup Caribbean Chicken and Rice, ½ cup green salad, 2 apricots.

EXERCISE: Rode my bike, Sebastian, to hair salon, post office, and grocery store. Played 1 hour ping pong with daughter and walked dog 2.5 miles.

TUESDAY

BREAKFAST: 1 egg, ½ slice buttered whole wheat toast, ½ cup yogurt

LUNCH 2 tablespoons of each: barley, quinoa, wheat berries, Red Lentils (1 tablespoon of each: kidney beans, garbanzo beans, great northern beans, black beans, fresh chopped red bell pepper, yellow bell pepper, green onion, Roma tomato, cilantro, and basil).

SNACK 1 tangelo and a 1-ounce slice of Gouda cheese

DINNER ¾ cup Chicken Cacciatore, 1 cup green salad, ½ cup steamed green beans

EXERCISE: Snow skiing and walked dog 1 mile.

WEDNESDAY

BREAKFAST 1 small Gingerbread Pancake brushed with syrup, 1 egg, ¾ cup milk

LUNCH ¾ cup Quinoa Salad and 1 tangelo

SNACK ½ cup green salad, ½ cup yogurt

DINNER 2 salmon patties, ½ cup wild rice, ½ cup green salad, ½ cup applesauce

EXERCISE: Rode Sebastian to post office and hardware store- 4 miles. Practiced yoga and walked dog 2.5 miles.

THURSDAY

BREAKFAST ½ cup quinoa, ½ teaspoon honey, ½ cup milk

LUNCH 2 tablespoons of each: barley, quinoa, wheat berries, Red Lentils (1 tablespoon of each: kidney beans, garbanzo beans, great northern beans, black beans, fresh chopped red bell pepper, yellow bell pepper, green onion, Roma tomato, cilantro, and basil).

SNACK Small handful (6 to 8) almonds and a grapefruit

DINNER 1 baked chicken thigh, ½ cup Rosemary Vegetable Bake, ½ cup green salad, 1 pear

EXERCISE: Rode Sebastian to an appointment in town 5 miles round trip. Weight training, played ping pong with son for 30 minutes, and walked dog 2.5 miles.

FRIDAY

BREAKFAST ¾ cup wheat berries and quinoa, ½ teaspoon honey, ½ cup milk

LUNCH 1 cup garbanzo beans in coconut milk and ½ slice Sourdough Whole Wheat Bread

SNACK ½ pomegranate, ½ cup yogurt

DINNER Takeout: ½ cup chicken chow mein over ⅓ cup rice noodles, 3 pieces of General Tso's chicken over ¼ cup rice

EXERCISE: Practiced yoga. Played 3 games of bowling with family and walked dog 2.5 miles

SATURDAY

BREAKFAST ¾ cup Wheat berries and quinoa, ½ teaspoon honey, ½ cup milk

LUNCH 2 tablespoons of each: barley, quinoa, wheat berries, Red Lentils (1 tablespoon of each: kidney beans, garbanzo beans, great northern beans, black beans, fresh chopped red bell pepper, yellow bell pepper, green onion, Roma tomato, cilantro, and basil).

SNACK 1 apple, small handful (6 to 8) almonds

DINNER 6-cheese ravioli with tomato basil sauce, ½ cup green salad

SNACK Exercise: Dancing—fox trot and swing—with husband for 1½ hours

SUNDAY

BREAKFAST 1 egg vegetable and cheese omelet (Green onions, cilantro, red and green bell peppers, diced tomatoes and ¼ cup Monterey Jack cheese, 1 cup milk, 1 Almond Pear Muffin

LUNCH ½ Pleasing Pita

SNACK 1 tangelo, ½ cup yogurt

DINNER ¾ cup spaghetti, ⅓ cup peas, 1 Spelt and Barley Bread Stick, ½ cup green salad, 1 peach

EXERCISE: Weight training, walked dog 2.5 miles, and 45 minutes ping pong with husband

MONDAY

BREAKFAST ½ cup cottage cheese with cucumbers, cilantro, chopped tomatoes and green onions, seasoned with flavor salt; 1 Sourdough Rye Muffin; 1 cup Spicy V8 juice

LUNCH 1 cup Carrot and Turnip Soup, 1 Sourdough Rye Muffin

SNACK ½ cup fresh mozzarella cheese, garden basil, and tomato slices drizzled with balsamic vinegar

DINNER 2 tablespoons of each: barley, quinoa, wheat berries and Red Lentils and 1 Apricot Cranberry Muffin

EXERCISE: Rode Sebastian for multiple errands around town, approximately 6 miles round trip, and walked dog 2.5 miles.

TUESDAY

BREAKFAST ¾ cup wheat berries and quinoa, ½ teaspoon honey, ½ cup milk

LUNCH 2 small Roasted Portabellas with Smoked Gouda and Fennel, 1 Apricot Cranberry Muffin

SNACK ½ cup green salad

DINNER Casablanca Chicken, ½ cup green salad, ½ cup stewed rhubarb

EXERCISE: Snow skiing

WEDNESDAY

BREAKFAST 1 egg, 1 Apple Spice Muffin, ½ cup yogurt

LUNCH ½ cup Jamaican Tofu with ½ cup rice

SNACK 1 cup popcorn lightly buttered and salted

DINNER ¾ cup sun-dried tomato pasta with chicken, ½ cup green salad, ¾ cup sautéed fresh spinach

EXERCISE: Yoga

THURSDAY

BREAKFAST 1 small Ginger Bread Pancake brushed with syrup, 1 scrambled egg, ¾ cup milk

LUNCH 1 cup Chipotle Pumpkin Soup and 1 Apple Spice Muffin

SNACK 1 cup Summer Delight Salad

DINNER 1 3-inch square serving of leftover lasagna, ½ cup green salad, ½ cup baked broccoli and cauliflower

EXERCISE: Weight training

FRIDAY

BREAKFAST ¾ cup Hot Millet Cereal with a few almonds and dates, 1 teaspoon honey, ½ cup milk

LUNCH 1 cup Lima Bean Vegetable Bowl

SNACK 1 peach

DINNER Shrimp Soup and Garlic French Bread

EXERCISE: None, movie night

SATURDAY

BREAKFAST ¾ cup steel-cut oats with raisins, 1 teaspoon honey, ½ cup milk

LUNCH 1 cup Lentil Skillet Dinner

SNACK 1 cup spinach salad

DINNER Ordered pizza: ½ slice of pizza with everything. ½ slice pepperoni pizza, 1 cup green salad, ½ grapefruit

EXERCISE: Hiking at Antelope Island

SUNDAY

BREAKFAST ¾ cup wheat berries and quinoa, ½ teaspoon honey, ½ cup milk

LUNCH 1 stuffed bell pepper

SNACK 2 apricots

DINNER Chicken Korma and flat bread with ½ cup mint, basil, and cilantro yogurt.

EXERCISE: Yoga and walked dog 2.5 miles.

TRENT'S W.O.W. DIET DIARY

In the summer of 2010, Trent asked if he could join me in the W.O.W. Diet. I was overjoyed to hear that Trent wanted to start eating more healthful foods. Upon further discussion, Trent disclosed that he wasn't so much interested in eating better but was motivated by the ease and sustainability of my weight loss.

Apparently, Trent had been experiencing back pain, and he believed it was due to being overweight. Trent said he saw the W.O.W. Diet as the ideal system for sustained weight loss because I ate inexpensive and delicious food, wasn't hungry between meals, and lost a significant amount of weight. I was a little disappointed in his response, but I admired his honesty. Either way, he would be eating healthy foods so I guess his motivation for going on the W.O.W. Diet didn't really matter.

I discussed having a conclusion in my book that would briefly track his journey in a diary format. He agreed. I wanted to take a picture of Trent with his shirt off, but he was embarrassed to have his pot belly recorded for the entire world to see. He did, however, agree to weekly weigh-ins and abdominal girth measurements. I measured his abdominal girth using his umbilicus as the measurement land mark. I measured him with the same measuring tape and at the same time of day each week. He measured his weight once a week, on the same calibrated scale, and at the same time of day.

I hope that readers find Trent's journey down the path of dietary enlightenment motivating and inspiring.

PERSONAL HISTORY

I am six feet tall, forty-seven years old, and weigh 208 pounds. I am about twenty pounds over-weight with the typical middle-age male paunch. I exercise lightly one to two times a week for thirty minutes and some weeks not at all. I have a desk job as an engineer. The only medication I take is Prevacid for acid reflux. I have had a lower back four level spinal fusion, and my extra weight is starting to cause pain in my lower back. Blood tests a year ago showed significant liver problems with enzyme levels of AST at 69 where the normal range is 15 to 40 and ALT at 119 where the normal range is 0 to 50.

RECENT PHYSICAL EXAMINATION RESULTS (JUST BEFORE THE DIET):

I am overweight by twenty to twenty-five pounds. My fatty-liver enzyme problem has not changed in a year (even though I did not spray chemicals around the yard, never drink alcoholic beverages, do not have hepatitis, or have a family history of liver problems). My blood pressure is borderline hypertensive (140/92); my cholesterol is reaching the higher range of normal: LDL of 133 where a normal range is 0 to 130 and cholesterol level of 196 where a normal range is 0 to 200.

STARTING COMMENTS

I personally feel that a target weight of 190 pounds with a belly-button girth of 35 inches would be a reasonable set point for me considering my age, genetics, and metabolism. I would like a set point I can easily maintain with enjoyable eating and moderate exercise. I plan to not change my exercise level during the diet until results are no longer noticeable by diet alone so as to not confound the results with other variables.

WEEK 1: LOST 2 INCHES AND 3½ POUNDS

Observations—I maintained my previous low level of exercise. I was only slightly hungry between meals; however, by eating a small healthy snack such as a piece of fruit, I did just fine. My overall GI system felt lighter and cleaner (not heavy and hard). My desired portion sizes decreased slightly around the third day. By Day 4, I noticed how much better and sweeter my fruit tasted. I also needed less honey to sweeten my whole grain cereal. If I was careful to eat regularly and consistently, I did not have any hunger, which was surprising to me. If I got caught up in work and forgot to eat regularly, I would get hungry and have a tendency to overeat at the next meal. I still like meat, but I desire less of it because my previous portions of meat made me feel "heavy" inside. In general, I really like how I am starting to feel "lighter and fresher" inside. My back pain has significantly reduced already.

WEEK 2: LOST ½ INCH AND 2 POUNDS

Observations—I maintained my previous level of exercise. I was not hungry between meals. I started craving the new foods over the old foods (I did have a *taste* of pizza and a few chips, but they did not feel satisfying). For breakfast I craved the new grains over the processed cereals. I do like an occasional egg for breakfast. I feel even better than I did the previous week. I feel lighter. I can walk a little faster and do a few extra pushups and so on. I have decided to start cutting back on my salt intake. My cheeks are less full and my double chin appears to be shrinking. My stool is consistently fluffy instead of hard.

WEEK 3: LOST ½ INCH AND 2 POUNDS

Observations—I was not hungry between meals. I continued to feel light inside and gain a little more energy. I am starting to see some of my upper stomach muscles that were previously buried in the belly fat.

WEEK 4: LOST ¼ INCH AND 1½ POUNDS

Observations—I maintained my previous level of exercise. I had two violations of the diet this week. Both proved very interesting. The first was when a good friend invited me over to celebrate her fortieth birthday and insisted I have ice cream and cake. I didn't want to offend her, so I ate the smallest piece of cake I could find and one small scoop of ice cream. The whole thing tasted "sickening" sweet. Within minutes, I had a sore throat (like an allergic reaction). I felt kind of sick for a couple of days afterward. The second occurrence was when another friend grilled T-bone steaks and had us over for dinner. Normally I eat moderate amounts of meat at only one meal a day. I ate the whole steak, just like I used to. My GI tract felt hard and heavy all night. If I would have stopped at half the steak and ate more vegetables, I am sure I would have felt great. I tend to desire healthy foods over processed foods now. I like how good I feel when I follow the diet.

WEEK 5: LOST 0 INCHES AND 0 POUNDS

Observations—Well, this was an interesting week. It appears that I am starting to plateau on the weight loss. I have reached half of my final set point goal in a month with diet change alone and no modi-fication to exercise. This week I only exercised once instead of my usual twice. Another difference is portion size. Although I did not violate the diet "types of foods," my wife has been busy writing and has not packed my "healthy" meals for work. Left to myself, I have packed more food than what I needed. The food tastes so good that I clean up my plate rather than stopping when I am full. I think the key to next week is to eat the right foods and the right portions and for now, maintain the usual low level of exercise. Bottom line, I feel much healthier eating these foods over the processed, high fat, high sugar foods. I also crave the new foods over the old foods. In no case have I felt hungry during this diet change.

WEEK 6: LOST 0 INCHES AND 1 POUND

Observations—This week was a little difficult because we went on a family road trip for five days. We were not able to cook, but I tried to eat healthy most times. No exercise except playing in the swimming pool and a short walk.

WEEK 7: LOST ¼ INCH AND 1 POUND

Observations—Back to the straight W.O.W. Diet this week. It is inter-esting that I am still losing weight even though I haven't increased my exercise. My stomach is somewhat flatter. My pants are all looser. I have even had to tighten my belt a notch or two. I am back down to a 34 pant waist! I am still curious to see where diet change alone will lead. I feel very healthy, and I am not hungry **if** I eat moderate portions on a regular basis throughout the day. Eating snacks of my favorite fruits or yogurt instead of sugars and junk food is one of the key points. If you do eat a processed desert, just taste, don't eat the whole thing. What I am saying is that it is important not to get hungry. Snacking is fine if you choose good snacks and eat in moderation.

WEEK 8: LOST ¼ INCH AND ½ POUNDS

Observations—I am starting to see some of my upper abdominal muscles that have been lost for some time. My back is not hurting like it used to. I think it is because I don't have as much weight on my spine.

WEEK 9: LOST 0 INCHES AND 1 POUND

Observations—I did pretty well on the diet this week, except one day when I went out to lunch with friends and ate Mexican food. I did not overeat to the extent I used to, but I did eat more than I needed to.

WEEK 10: LOST ¼ INCH AND 1 POUND

Observations—I was not perfect with the diet this week. My wife was out of town, and I did not make grains and so forth. I ate some commercial cereal, sandwiches, and 1 piece of pizza. I only exercised one day.

WEEK 11: LOST 0 INCHES AND 1 POUND

Observations—Pretty much stuck to the diet.

WEEK 12 – LOST 0 INCHES AND GAINED ½ POUND

Observations—I only exercised one day. Stuck to the W.O.W. Diet except my wife made pound cake for dinner guests, and I had a small slice here and there. My proportions were pretty much per the diet.

PARTING THOUGHTS

Having been on the W.O.W. Diet for 12 weeks, I have lost a total of 14 pounds and 5 inches. As of September 2010, my liver enzymes have dropped from a harmful AST of 69 to a healthier 34. My ALT has also decreased from a dangerously high 119 to a nearly normal range of 51. I can't believe the difference in how I feel and how I am not hungry yet I am losing weight!

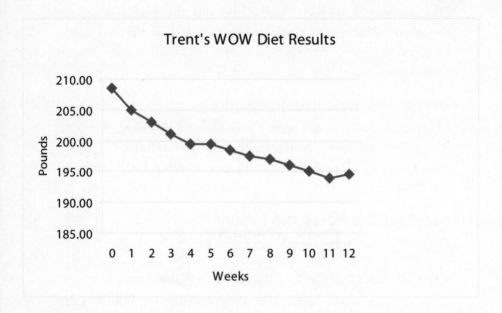

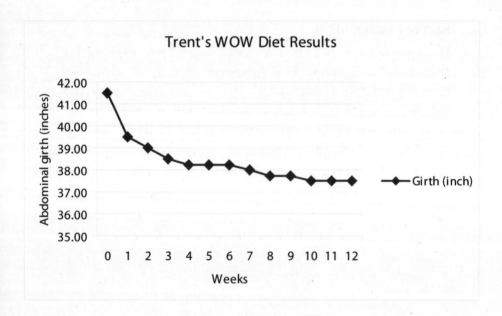

APPENDIX A:

RECIPES

(GLUTEN FREE RECIPES ARE MARKED "GF")

ALMOND COCONUT PANCAKES (GF)

1¼ cups water

2 eggs

1½ cups almond flour

½ cup gluten-free oat flour

½ cup millet flour

½ tsp. salt

1 tsp. baking soda

2 tsp. almond extract

3 Tbsp. honey

2 Tbsp. oil

1 cup angel flake coconut

In a large bowl, stir together all ingredients except coconut flakes until batter is smooth. Gently stir in coconut. Ladle pancake batter onto a hot oiled griddle. Turn pancakes when bubbles appear and edges are golden brown. **Note:** You must use a thin spatula to quickly slide and flip the pancakes because they're so delicate. No syrup is needed for these amazing pancakes!

PANCAKES (GF)

1½ cups milk

½ cup water

2 cups millet flour

1 cup amaranth flour

2 tsp. baking powder

2 Tbsp. granulated white sugar

1 tsp. salt

2 eggs

¼ cup canola oil

½ tsp. vanilla extract

In a large bowl, mix together all ingredients until smooth. Ladle batter onto a hot oiled griddle. Turn pancakes when bubbles appear and edges are golden brown.

GINGERBREAD PANCAKES (GF)

¾ cup water

1 cup amaranth flour

¼ tsp. salt

3 Tbsp. brown sugar

½ tsp. ground cinnamon

⅛ tsp. ground cloves

⅓ cup powdered milk

1 egg

1 tsp. baking powder

1 Tbsp. oil

In a large bowl, mix together all ingredients until smooth. Ladle batter onto a hot oiled griddle. Turn pancakes when bubbles appear and edges are golden brown.

BUCKWHEAT PANCAKES (GF)

3 cups buckwheat flour

4 cups buttermilk

3 eggs

3 Tbsp. oil

2 tsp. baking powder

1 tsp. baking soda

1 tsp. salt

3 Tbsp. granulated white sugar

1 pkg. chocolate chips (optional)

In a large bowl, stir together all ingredients until batter is smooth. Ladle pancake batter onto a hot oiled griddle. Turn pancakes when bubbles appear.

BUTTERMILK CHOCOLATE CHIP PANCAKES (GF)

1¼ cups buttermilk

1 cup rice flour

2 eggs

6 Tbsp. millet flour

⅔ cup oat flour

2 Tbsp. white sugar

1½ tsp. baking powder

½ tsp. salt

1 tsp. vanilla

½ cup mini chocolate chips

In a large bowl, stir together all ingredients except chocolate chips until smooth. Fold in chocolate chips. Ladle pancake batter onto a hot oiled griddle. Turn pancakes when bubbles appear and edges are golden brown.

WHOLE WHEAT PANCAKES WITH BUTTERMILK AND EGGS

(Original recipe from the kitchen of my
mother-in-law, Rosalie Snow)

3 cups wheat flour

3 cups buttermilk

3 eggs

3 Tbsp. oil

2 tsp. baking powder

1 tsp. baking soda

1 tsp. salt

3 Tbsp. granulated white sugar

In a large bowl, stir together all ingredients until batter is smooth. Ladle pancake batter onto a hot oiled griddle. Turn pancakes when bubbles appear and edges are golden brown.

POTATO CORNMEAL PANCAKES (GF)

2 cups milk

1 cup water

½ cup potato flour

1 cup cornmeal

1 tsp. granulated white sugar

2 eggs

¼ tsp. salt

1 tsp. baking soda

In a large bowl, stir together all ingredients until smooth. Ladle batter onto a hot oiled griddle. Turn pancakes when bubbles appear and edges are golden brown.

NIGHT BEFORE APPLE RAISIN STRATA

This is not healthy, but it is so delicious I had to share it.

1 loaf raisin cinnamon bread or day-old French bread,
  cut into cubes

1 (8-oz.) package cream cheese

1 cup raisins

3–4 tart green apples, peeled, cored, and sliced

1 quart half and half

8 eggs

½ teaspoon salt

Cinnamon and sugar

Maple syrup (optional)

Butter a 9 x 13 baking dish. Spread half of bread cubes evenly in baking dish, covering completely. Slice cream cheese and place on top of bread cubes. Sprinkle with raisins. Arrange apple slices over raisins. Top apple layer with remaining bread cubes. In a medium-sized bowl, whisk half and half, eggs, and salt. Add cinnamon, varying amounts based on desired sweetness. Gently pour mixture over bread cubes. Allow strata to chill overnight. In the morning, preheat oven to 350°F. Bake for 30–45 minutes or until egg is set. For added sweetness, drizzle strata with pure maple syrup before serving.

HOT BARLEY CEREAL

6 cups water

1½ cups barley

Brown sugar

Nuts

Dried fruit

Milk

In a heavy saucepan with a tight-fitting lid, simmer water and barley for 1 hour over low heat. Serve with sugar, nuts, or dried fruit and milk to taste.

CRACKED WHEAT CEREAL

3 cups water

1 cup cracked wheat

Milk

Brown sugar

In heavy saucepan with a tight-fitting lid, simmer water and barley for 1 hour over low heat. Serve with sugar, nuts, or dried fruit and milk to taste.

BREAKFAST COUSCOUS

2 cups water

2 Tbsp. honey

3 tsp. ground cinnamon

2 cups couscous

⅓ cup dried apricots

⅓ cup raisins

½ cup sliced almonds

Milk

In a medium saucepan over medium-high heat, combine water, honey, and cinnamon. When water reaches a boil, stir in couscous. Remove from heat, cover, and let stand for 5 minutes. Add apricots, raisins, and almonds. Serve with milk to taste.

QUINOA (GF)

1½ cups water

1 cup quinoa

Sugar

Nuts

Dried fruit

Milk

In a heavy saucepan* over medium heat, combine water and quinoa. Bring water and quinoa to a boil, stirring occasionally. Reduce heat to medium-low and simmer for 20 minutes or until quinoa is soft. To serve, add sugar, nuts, or dried fruit and milk to taste.

*I prefer to cook my quinoa in a rice cooker.

HOT TEFF CEREAL (GF)

½ cup teff, toasted

2 cups water

Milk

Brown sugar

Cinnamon

Nuts

Dried fruit

Coconut

In a medium pan, combine teff and water. Bring to boil over medium heat, stirring frequently. Cook for 20 minutes or until water is absorbed. Add milk, brown sugar, cinnamon, nuts, dried fruit, or coconut to taste.

HOT 6-GRAIN CEREAL

6 cups water

4 cups 6-grain cereal

Sugar

Nuts

Dried fruit

Milk

In a medium saucepan over high heat, bring water to a rolling boil. Reduce heat to medium and add cereal. Cook cereal until soft, 25 to 30 minutes, stirring occasionally. To serve, add sugar, nuts, or dried fruit and milk to taste.

HOT MILLET CEREAL (GF)

1 cup cracked millet

¾ cup powdered milk

4 cups water

Dried fruit

Nuts

Brown sugar

Milk

Process millet in blender until it reaches the consistency of uncooked cream of wheat. In a medium saucepan, combine powdered milk and water. Bring to a boil over medium heat. Add cracked millet, stirring continuously. Cook for 5 minutes or until thickened. Add fruits, nuts, brown sugar, and milk to taste.

BROWN RICE BREAKFAST (GF)

(Original recipe from the kitchen of Ann Stanger)

3 cups cooked brown rice

3 cups milk

1¼ tsp. ground cinnamon

5 Tbsp. raisins

4 tsp. chopped nuts

¾ cup maple syrup

Warm all ingredients in a small saucepan over medium heat.

RICE PUDDING (GF)

2 cups water

1 cup brown rice

2 cups milk

½ cup granulated white sugar

¼ cup raisins

1 tsp. ground cinnamon

1 tsp. orange zest

3 Tbsp. sweetened coconut.

Cook rice: In a heavy-bottomed saucepan with a tight-fitting lid, bring water and rice to a boil over high heat and cook for 15 minutes. Remove from heat and set aside for 10 minutes. Do not lift lid and peek at the rice while it is resting! Fluff rice with fork. If you have a rice cooker, just add water and rice and press the lever. Fluff rice when lever pops up.

Combine remaining ingredients in a medium saucepan and cook for 30 minutes over low heat, stirring frequently. Rice pudding may be served warm or cold.

CHOCOLATE CHIP MUFFINS (GF)

Vegetable shortening

¾ cup rice flour

½ cup oat flour

¼ cup tapioca flour

¼ cup brown sugar

1 tsp. baking soda

½ tsp. salt

2 Tbsp. powdered milk

2 Tbsp. powdered eggs

½ cup water

½ cup melted butter, cooled

2 tsp. vanilla extract

1 cup chocolate chips

½ cup coarsely chopped almonds

Preheat oven to 375°F. Grease muffin pan cups with vegetable shortening. In a large bowl, combine dry ingredients, leaving a well in the center. Stir in water, melted butter, and vanilla until moist. Fold in chocolate chips and nuts. Spoon batter into muffin cups. Bake for 20 minutes or until a toothpick inserted into the middle of a muffin comes out clean. Cool muffins 5 minutes before removing from cups.

PUMPKIN MUFFINS (GF)

Vegetable shortening

1 cup canned pumpkin puree

¾ cup water

¾ cup amaranth flour

½ cup flaxseed meal

¼ cup quinoa flour

1 Tbsp. baking powder

1¼ tsp. pumpkin pie spice

½ tsp. baking soda

½ tsp. salt

⅓ cup powdered milk

1 egg

1 cup raisins (My children request chocolate chips instead. I give in on occasion.)

⅓ cup oil

½ cup honey

Preheat oven to 400°F. Grease muffin pan cups with vegetable shortening. In a large bowl, mix together all ingredients until moist. Fill muffin cups two-thirds full of batter. Bake 20 to 25 minutes or until a toothpick inserted into the center of a muffin comes out clean. Cool muffins 5 minutes before removing from cups.

APPLE SPICE MUFFINS (GF)

1½ cup cooked quinoa

1½ cup amaranth flour

½ cup millet flour

½ cup quinoa flour

2 cups water

¼ cup safflower oil

2 eggs

½ cup brown sugar

½ cup honey

1 Tbsp. vanilla

1 tsp. cinnamon

1 tsp. baking soda

1½ tsp. baking powder

¾ tsp. salt

1 cup green apple, chopped

1 cup raisins

Vegetable shortening for muffin cups or muffin cup
   liners

Preheat oven to 375°F. In a large bowl, combine all ingredients except apples and raisins and stir until blended. Fold in apple and raisins. Grease muffin cups or fill muffin cup liners two-thirds full. Bake for 20–22 minutes. Muffins are done when a toothpick inserted into the middle comes out clean. These muffins freeze well.

ITALIANO MILLET MUFFINS (GF)

2 Tbsp. Italian seasonings

½ tsp. baking powder

½ tsp. salt

¼ tsp. onion powder

⅓ cup coarsely grated Parmesan cheese

¾ cup millet flour

¾ cup amaranth flour

2 eggs

1 cup Parmesan cheese

1 cup buttermilk

¼ cup water

¼ cup oil

Vegetable shortening for muffin cups or muffin cup liners

Preheat oven to 375°F. Mix dry ingredients and form a well. Stir in liquids and mix just until batter is moist. Grease muffin cups or use muffin cup liners. Fill cups three-fourths full and bake for 20–25 minutes. Muffins are done when a toothpick inserted into the middle comes out clean.

ALMOND PEAR MUFFIN (GF)

1 cup teff flour

1¼ cups amaranth flour

¼ cup flax meal

1½ tsp. baking powder

1¼ tsp. baking soda

1 tsp. salt

½ tsp. ground ginger

1 cup buttermilk

2 eggs

2 cups pears (fresh or canned)

½ cup butter

½ cup honey

1 tsp. almond extract

¾ cup sliced almonds

Vegetable shortening for muffin cups or muffin liners

Preheat oven to 375°F. Mix dry ingredients and form a well. Stir in liquids until batter is moist. Fold in sliced almonds. Grease muffin cups or use muffin cup liners. Fill cups three-fourths full and bake for 20–25 minutes. Muffins are done when a toothpick inserted into the middle comes out clean.

BRAN MUFFIN

¾ cup water

3 Tbsp. cooled melted butter

1 cup whole wheat flour

3 Tbsp. granulated white sugar

1 egg

3½ tsp. baking powder

¼ tsp. salt

3 Tbsp. milk

1 cup bran

Vegetable shortening for muffin cups or muffin cup
    liners

Preheat oven to 400°F. Grease muffin cups or use muffin cup liners. In a medium bowl, mix all ingredients until moist. Fill muffin cups two thirds full of batter. Bake for 20 to 25 minutes or until a toothpick inserted into the center of a muffin comes out clean. Cool muffins 5 minutes before removing from cups.

APRICOT CRANBERRY MUFFINS

1 cup oat flour

1½ cups whole wheat flour

1 cup oats

1 cup white granulated sugar

1½ tsp. baking powder

1¼ tsp. baking soda

½ tsp. salt

¾ cup canned apricots, drained and pureed

3 Tbsp. oil

2 eggs

1¾ cup canned apricots, mashed

1 cup dried cranberries

1 cup white chocolate chips, *optional* (too sweet for me
   to eat, but the rest of the family likes this addition)

Vegetable shortening for muffin cups or muffin cup
   liners

Preheat oven to 375°F. Place dry ingredients in a large bowl and stir. Place ¾ cup canned apricots, oil, and eggs in blender and process until pureed. Pour blended mixture into dry ingredients and stir until mixed. Add mashed apricots. Stir in dried cranberries and white chocolate chips. Grease muffin cups or use muffin tin liners. Fill cups two thirds full and bake for 20–25 minutes. Muffins are done when a toothpick inserted into the middle comes out clean.

SOURDOUGH RYE MUFFINS

2 cups sourdough start

1 cup rye flour

1 egg, beaten

2 Tbsp. oil

3 Tbsp. honey

1 Tbsp. baking powder

½ tsp. salt

¼ cup yogurt

Vegetable shortening for muffin cups or muffin cup
    liners

Preheat oven to 400°F. In a medium mixing bowl, mix all ingredients except yogurt. Once batter is moist, stir in yogurt until just mixed into batter. Grease muffin cups or use muffin cup liners. Fill muffin cups two-thirds full with batter. Bake for 20–25 minutes or until a toothpick inserted into the middle of a muffin comes out clean.

OAT CRUMB CAKE MUFFINS (GF)

Topping:

  ⅓ cup softened canned butter

  ¼ cup rice flour

  ¼ cup gluten-free oat flour

  ⅔ cup gluten-free oats

  ⅓ cup brown sugar

  ½ tsp. cinnamon

Batter:

  ¾ cup rice flour

  ½ cup gluten-free oat flour

  ¼ cup tapioca flour

  ½ cup granulated white sugar

  1 tsp. baking soda

  ½ tsp. salt

  2 Tbsp. powdered egg

  2 Tbsp. powdered milk

  ½ cup water

  ½ cup cooled melted canned butter

  1 tsp. vanilla extract

  ½ tsp. almond extract

  vegetable shortening

Preheat oven to 375°F. In a small bowl, combine topping ingredients until they resemble small crumbs. Pour dry ingredients into a large bowl and form a well. Add water, butter, vanilla, and almond extract. Stir just enough to combine dry ingredients with the wet ingredients. Do not over mix. Grease muffin pan cups with vegetable shortening. Fill muffin cups two-thirds full of batter. Top muffin batter with prepared topping. Bake for 20 to 25 minutes or until a toothpick inserted into the middle of a muffin comes out clean. Cool muffins 5 minutes before removing from cups.

Tip: Use the muffin topping for a quick and delicious gluten-free cobbler topping.

WHOLE WHEAT FRENCH BREAD

2¼ tsp. yeast

1 cup whole wheat flour

1½–2½ cups bread flour

1 Tbsp. sugar

2 tsp. salt

1½ cups warm water

Egg Wash

1 egg and 3 Tbsp. water whisked together

Preheat oven to 400°F. Mix yeast, whole wheat flour, 1½ cups bread flour, sugar, and salt in a large bowl. Add water. If dough is too wet, gradually add more bread flour. You may not need to use all of the flour. Knead dough on a lightly floured counter, adding flour until dough is no longer sticky. Place dough in a large oiled bowl and cover with plastic wrap. Let rise until doubled in size. Turn out dough onto floured surface and shape as desired. Transfer dough onto an oiled cookie sheet that has been sprinkled with cornmeal or onto a French bread loaf pan. Allow to rise until loaf has doubled in size. Brush top with egg wash and bake for 30–35 minutes.

PUMPERNICKEL BREAD

7 tsp. yeast

1½ cups warm water

4 tsp. salt

½ cup molasses

2 Tbsp. caraway seeds

2¾ cups rye flour

3–3½ cups bread flour

2 Tbsp. vegetable shortening, melted

1 cup boiling water

Place a pie tin on bottom rack of oven. Preheat oven to 450°F. In a large bowl, mix yeast, water, salt, molasses and caraway seeds. Combine flours in separate bowl. Add half of flour to liquids and stir. Blend, adding flour as needed until dough is no longer sticky. Place dough on lightly floured counter and knead for 10 minutes. Move dough to an oiled bowl. Cover bowl with a damp cloth and place in a warm spot. When dough has doubled in size (takes about 2 hours), punch down and cut into 2 halves. Shape dough into round, smooth balls. Place on a cookie sheet lightly dusted with cornmeal. Cover with damp cloth and allow to rise for 30–40 minutes. Spritz loaves with water and place in oven. Fill pie tin with 1 cup boiling water. Bake at 450° for 10 minutes. Reduce heat to 350° and bake for 25 more minutes.

SPELT AND BARLEY BREAD STICKS

2 cups warm water

⅔ cup powdered milk

2 Tbsp. yeast

¼ cup sugar

2 tsp. salt

⅓ cup butter melted

1 egg

4–4½ cups spelt flour

1 cup barley flour

Your choice cheese, onions, or seeds

Preheat oven to 375°F. In a large bowl, combine all ingredients except flours. Mix flours in a separate bowl. Add half of flour mixture and stir until well mixed. Add flour until dough is not sticky. You may not need to use all of the flour. Knead dough for 3 minutes. Move dough to a large oiled bowl. Cover bowl with plastic wrap. Allow bread to rise until doubled in size. Place dough on a lightly floured counter and shape as desired. Move to an oiled cookie sheet and allow to rise for 30 minutes. Brush bread sticks with egg wash and sprinkle with desired cheeses, onions, or seeds. Bake for 10 minutes.

SOURDOUGH ROSEMARY BREAD

2 cups sourdough starter (I allow mine to bubble 3 days
    for extra tanginess.)

¼ cup olive oil

2 tsp. yeast

2 tsp. salt

2 Tbsp. rosemary

2–3½ cups bread flour

1 cup boiling water

Place a pie tin on the bottom rack. Preheat oven to 450°F. In a large bag, mix sourdough starter, olive oil, yeast, salt, rosemary, and half of flour. Mix thoroughly with a spoon. Add flour until dough is tender but not sticky. You may not need all of the flour. Knead dough for 3 minutes. Place in an oiled bowl, cover with plastic wrap, and allow to rise until doubled. Remove from bowl and shape as desired. Allow to rise on a cornmeal sprinkled baking stone or cookie sheet for 30–40 minutes. Spritz with water and place in oven on center rack. Immediately add 1 cup boiling water to pie tin and quickly close oven. Bake until crust is browned and loaf sounds hollow when tapped, usually 35–45 minutes.

SOURDOUGH WHOLE WHEAT BREAD

2 cups sourdough starter

1¼ tsp. yeast

½ cup honey

2½ tsp. salt

1 cup warm water

1 cup yogurt

4 cups whole wheat flour

2–3 cups bread flour

Preheat oven to 350°F. In a large bowl, combine all of the ingredients except flour. Add whole wheat flour and stir. Add bread flour until dough is tender but not sticky. Knead for 10 minutes on a lightly floured surface. Place in an oiled bowl, cover with plastic wrap, and let rise until doubled. Remove from bowl. Divide dough in half, shape loaves as desired, and place in greased bread pans. Bake for 45–55 minutes or until crust is brown and loaf sounds hollow when tapped. Lightly spritz with water for a softer crust immediately after removing baked loaves from the oven.

PLEASING PITAS

Bean Salad

1 (15.5-oz.) can kidney beans, drained and rinsed

1 (15-oz.) can butter beans, drained and rinsed

1 (14-oz.) can cannellini beans, drained and rinsed

1 (14-oz.) can artichoke hearts, drained and rinsed

4 Tbsp. prepared quinoa

4 Tbsp. prepared barley pearls

4 Tbsp. wheat berries

4 Tbsp. lentils

1 red bell pepper, chopped

½ cup chopped Anaheim pepper

1 medium red onion, finely chopped

½ bunch cilantro, chopped

Dressing:

¾ cup sweet chili sauce

½ cup olive oil

2 Tbsp. granulated white sugar

1 lemon, juiced

1 package whole wheat pita bread

Condiments:

Avocado slices

Tomato slices

Sprouts

Place salad ingredients in bowl. Prepare dressing and pour over bean salad. Toss until salad is coated in dressing. Carefully slice 1 piece of pita bread in half and fill with bean salad and desired condiments. Complete your meal with a side of mixed fruit.

GARDEN SHELLS

2 tsp. minced garlic

1 small yellow onion, finely chopped

2 Tbsp. olive oil

2 cups chopped broccoli

3 medium carrots, shredded

2 cups fresh spinach leaves

¼ cup fresh basil, chopped

2 Tbsp. fresh oregano, chopped

1 cup ricotta cheese or cottage cheese

1 (12-oz.) package jumbo pasta shells, cooked
   according to instructions

1–2 cups marinara sauce

¾ cup mozzarella cheese, shredded

3 Tbsp. grated Romano cheese

Preeat oven to 350°F In a large skillet over medium-high heat, sauté garlic and onions in olive oil. Add broccoli and carrots and sauté until tender. Add spinach, basil, and oregano. Cook for 3–5 minutes until spinach is tender. Place cooked vegetables in a bowl to cool. Once vegetables have cooled, add ricotta cheese and mix. Spoon vegetable filling into prepared pasta shells. Place filled shells on an oiled baking dish. Ladle marinara sauce over filled shells and top with mozzarella cheese followed by a sprinkling of Romano cheese. Bake for 30 minutes.

LIMA BEAN VEGETABLE BOWL (GF)

1 tsp. garlic

2 Tbsp. safflower oil

½ cup chopped white onion

1 cup sliced zucchini

1 sliced yellow squash

1 cup chopped watercress

1 cup cooked quinoa

½ cup lima beans

2 large fresh tomatoes, cubed

Salt and pepper to taste

¼ cup Parmesan cheese

In a large skillet, sauté garlic in oil over medium-high heat. Add zucchini, squash, and watercress. When vegetables are partially cooked and almost tender, add watercress. When vegetables are tender, add quinoa and lima beans. Top with fresh tomatoes, salt and pepper, and Parmesan cheese.

SPINACH SALAD

2 cups fresh spinach

¼ cup mandarin oranges

2 Tbsp. fresh or dried cranberries

2 Tbsp. fresh or dried blueberries

2 Tbsp. fresh sliced strawberries

2 Tbsp. blue cheese crumbles

2 Tbsp. Chow Mein noodles

1 Tbsp. sesame seeds

1 Tbsp. pumpkin seeds

1 Tbsp. sunflower seeds

Wash spinach leaves and pat dry. Toss in remaining ingredients. Serve with Poppy Seed Dressing (see page 135).

POPPY SEED DRESSING (GF)

1 cup granulated white sugar

⅔ cup rice vinegar

¼ cup chopped red onion

3 tsp. dry mustard

1 tsp. salt

2 cups safflower oil

2 Tbsp. poppy seeds

Combine first five ingredients in a blender. Process ingredients on medium speed until well blended. With blender on a low speed, drizzle oil into mixture. Dressing will become thick and creamy. Once oil is incorporated, stir in poppy seeds. Refrigerate any unused portion in a sealed container.

STUFFED BELL PEPPERS (GF)

½ cup yellow onion, chopped

2 tsp. minced garlic

½ cup celery, sliced

2 Tbsp. oil

2 cups cooked quinoa

1 cup jicama

½ cup cilantro, chopped

4 bell peppers

1 cup Chipotle Sauce (see below)

4 parsley sprigs, chopped

Preheat oven to 350°F. In a small saucepan, cook onions, garlic, and celery in oil until tender. In a large bowl, mix onions, garlic, and celery with quinoa and jicama. Remove tops from bell peppers and scrape out seeds and membranes until hollow. Fill bell pepper with quinoa filling. Place bell peppers upright in a 9 x 9 pan and bake at 350° for 35–45 minutes. Place ¼ cup Chipotle Sauce in the center of a dinner plate and sprinkle with fresh chopped parsley. Carefully place stuffed bell pepper in the center of the chipotle sauce and serve.

CHIPOTLE SAUCE (GF)

3 chipotle peppers in adobo sauce

1¼ cup plain yogurt

1 lime, juiced

Place all ingredients in blender and process until smooth. Refrigerate in an airtight container.

SANTA FE BURRITO

Tortillas

1 cup quinoa

1½ cups water

1 (14-oz.) can firm tofu, cubed

1 Tbsp. safflower oil

1 tsp. minced garlic

4 Tbsp. Chipotle Sauce (see page 136) or BBQ sauce

1 large avocado, sliced

4 green onions, chopped

1 cup jicama, julienned

1 can black beans, drained

1 can corn, drained

1 medium tomato, diced

1 medium cucumber sliced

1 cup alfalfa sprouts

¼ cup Anaheim pepper

In a heavy-bottomed sauce pan with a tight-fitting lid, add 1 cup quinoa to 1 cup water. Boil on high heat for 15 minutes. Remove from heat and set aside for 10 minutes, then fluff. Do not lift the lid and peek at the quinoa while it is resting. If you have a rice cooker, just add water and quinoa and press the lever. Fluff quinoa when lever pops up.

Drain tofu and cube. In a small pan, heat oil and fry garlic and tofu until lightly browned. Remove tofu and cut into cubes. Toss tofu cubes in chipotle sauce. Warm tortilla in microwave for 10 seconds. Place desired ingredients in tortilla and serve. Complete your meal with a side of apple and orange slices.

STICK RICE NOODLE SALAD (GF)

1 (10.75-oz.) package stick rice noodles or
    rice vermicelli (green mung bean noodles
    may be substituted)
1 cup matchstick carrots
2 stalks celery, sliced
5 green onions, chopped
1 cup pea pods
1 cup cilantro, chopped
½ cup water chestnuts, chopped
1 cup vegetable or chicken broth
2 Tbsp. brown sugar
1 Tbsp. white sugar
4 limes, juiced
1½ tsp. fish sauce (check lable; some are made with
    wheat proteins)
½ tsp. chili garlic sauce
Chopped peanuts

Cook noodles according to directions on package. While noodles are cooking, mix together remaining ingredients and prepare vegetables. When noodles are tender, rinse and drain according to package directions and toss with vegetables and chili garlic sauce. Garnish with chopped peanuts and serve.

PAD THAI

2 cups cubed chicken breast

3 Tbsp. oil

1 tsp. minced garlic

6 cups water

1 (10.75-oz.) package stick rice noodles or
    rice vermicelli (green mung bean noodles
    may be substituted)

Pad Thai sauce (we like the Por Kwan brand)

½ cup chopped peanuts

½ cup fresh chopped cilantro

In a large skillet over medium-high heat, cook chicken breast in oil and garlic. In a large saucepan, bring water to a rolling boil. Place noodles in boiling water and cook 5–8 minutes. Drain noodles and rinse with cool water. Gently toss chicken and noodles with just enough Pad Thai sauce to coat noodles. Transfer noodles to serving platter. Top with chopped peanuts and fresh cilantro.

THAI LETTUCE WRAPS (GF)

1 pound beef, chicken, or shrimp cut into ¼ by 2-inch strips

2 Tbsp. vegetable oil

1 tsp. minced garlic

1 cup shredded Napa cabbage

½ cup matchstick carrots

1 (6-oz.) can water chestnuts, chopped

1 cup prepared brown rice

2 Tbsp. mint leaves, chopped

3 Tbsp. cilantro, chopped

¼ cup chopped green onion

¾ cup sweet Thai chili sauce

¾ cup peanuts, chopped

12 Bibb lettuce leaves

2 limes, sliced

In a large pan, cook meat in oil and garlic. When meat is thoroughly cooked, add cabbage, carrots and water chestnuts. Cook 5 minutes or until cabbage is tender. Stir in rice, mint, cilantro, green onion, sweet Thai chili sauce, and peanuts. Place a washed and dried lettuce leaf on each plate and spoon about ½ cup mixture in the center of each leaf. Squeeze lime over filling and serve.

VEGETARIAN TOSTADA (GF)

Hummus:

 1 (14.5-oz.) can garbanzo beans, rinsed and drained,
     reserving liquid
 4 tsp. fresh lemon juice
 2 tsp. minced garlic
 ¼ tsp. salt
 Cayenne pepper to taste

1 box cornmeal tostada shells

Toppings:

 Sprouts
 Roma tomatoes, chopped
 Assorted peppers, such as bell, Anaheim, or jalapeño
 Black olives, sliced
 Green onions, chopped
 Pepper jack cheese, goat cheese, or queso fresco
     cheese
 Black beans, rinsed and drained
 Avocado slices

In a blender or food processor, combine all hummus
ingredients, adding reserved liquid to reach a medium
thick consistency.
Spoon 1–2 tablespoons hummus on a tostada shell and
add desired toppings.

PARSNIP SOUP (GF)

2 cups vegetable or chicken broth

6 parsnips, cut into ¼ inch slices

¼ tsp. garam marsala

¼ tsp. ginger

1 cup milk

1 cup prepared lentils

1 Tbsp. chopped green onions

3 Tbsp. finely chopped fresh parsley

In a large saucepan over medium heat, combine broth, parsnips, garam marsala, and ginger and cook until parsnips are tender. Transfer parsnip mixture and milk to blender and puree until smooth. Stir in lentils, green onions, and parsley. If you are gluten intolerant, be sure to use a gluten-free broth.

VEGETARIAN SPAGHETTI (GF)

1 spaghetti squash

1 cup sliced mushrooms

1 medium-sized eggplant, cubed

1 zucchini, sliced

1 green bell pepper, sliced

1 medium white onion, chopped

1 tsp. minced garlic

2 Tbsp. olive oil

1 bottle marinara sauce

½ cup Parmesan cheese

Preheat oven to 350°F. Cut squash and clean out seeds. Bake squash in preheated oven at 350° for 45 minutes or until squash is tender. In a medium-sized pan, sauté remaining vegetables and garlic in oil until tender. Toss vegetables in marinara sauce. Once squash is tender, run a fork back and forth along squash flesh until flesh resembles spaghetti. Discard squash shell. Place spaghetti squash on a platter and top with vegetable marinara sauce. Garnish with Parmesan cheese. Serve with Whole Wheat French Bread (see page 126) or Spelt and Barley Bread Sticks (Page 128).

VEGETABLES IN LEMON CAPER SAUCE (GF)

1 heaping tsp. minced garlic

2 Tbsp. olive oil

1 cup sliced mushrooms

1 cup eggplant

1 zucchini

1 yellow squash

1 cup chicken breast, cubed (optional)

⅛ tsp. white pepper

1 (14-oz.) can artichoke hearts, drained

Sauce

3 cups vegetable or chicken broth

2 Tbsp. washed capers

2 tsp. arrowroot or cornstarch

¼ cup water

juice of ½ lemon

4 cups cooked quinoa

Garnish

¼ cup yellow bell pepper,

¼ cup red bell pepper

2 Tbsp. green onion

2 Tbsp. chopped rosemary

¼ cup fresh chopped basil

⅛ tsp. white pepper

In a large skillet, sauté garlic and oil over medium high heat. Add vegetables and, if desired, cubed chicken. Season with white pepper and cook vegetables until tender. Add artichoke hearts.

In a medium saucepan, simmer broth and capers for 10 minutes. Combine arrowroot and water in small bowl and stir until smooth. Add arrowroot mixture to broth, stirring until sauce achieves desired thickness. Add juice of ½ lemon. Pour lemon caper sauce over vegetables and toss. Place cooked quinoa on platter, followed by vegetable mixture. Garnish and serve. If you are gluten intolerant be sure to use a gluten free bouillon.

GARBANZO BEANS IN COCONUT MILK (GF)

3 cups water

2 cups rice

2 (15-oz.) cans garbanzo beans*, including juice

1 (13.5-oz.) can coconut milk

2 cups Roma tomatoes

½ cup cilantro, chopped

½ tsp. garam masala

½ tsp. powdered coriander

1 tsp. garlic powder

1 tsp. turmeric

2 tsp. curry powder

1 Tbsp. granulated white sugar

¼ tsp. cayenne pepper

In a heavy-bottomed saucepan with a tight-fitting lid, boil rice and water on high heat for 15 minutes or until tender. Remove from heat and set aside for 10 minutes and then fluff. Do not lift the lid and peek at the rice while it is resting! If you have a rice cooker, just add water and rice and press the lever. Fluff rice when lever pops up.

In a large saucepan combine garbanzo beans, coconut milk, tomatoes, cilantro, and spices. Simmer over medium heat for 10 minutes. To serve, spoon garbanzo bean mixture over rice. Complete your meal with homemade yogurt and fresh blueberries.

* Garbanzo beans and chickpeas are different names for the same bean.

CARROT AND TURNIP SOUP (GF)

4 small turnips, cubed

¼ cup butter

1 medium white onion, chopped

2 tsp. garlic, minced

4 cups chicken or vegetable broth

7 large carrots, sliced

1 cup milk

1 cup fresh cilantro, chopped

Salt and pepper to taste

Place cubed turnips in pan and cover with water. Boil turnips until tender. Remove from burner and drain water. Place butter, onion, and garlic in skillet and cook until onions start turning translucent. Add broth and carrots and cook at a rolling boil until carrots turn soft. Add milk. Place carrot mixture in food processor and blend until smooth. Stir in turnips and cilantro and serve. If you are gluten intolerant, be sure to use a gluten-free broth.

YOGURT (GF)

(Original recipe from the kitchen of Tammy Hulse)

(Makes 1 gallon yogurt)

1 gallon 2 percent or whole milk*

½ cup powdered milk

1 cup plain yogurt

Sweetener of choice**

Probiotics, if desired

Preheat oven on warm setting. Place milk and powdered milk in a large, heavy-bottomed stainless steel stock pot and heat to 180°F, stirring often. Turn off oven and turn on oven light. Once milk has reached 180°, cool to 125–110°F. (I place the pot in a sink full of ice water; within 5 to 10 minutes the milk is cooled.) Stir in yogurt, sweetener, and probiotics if desired. Pour into pint-sized canning jars and cover with a canning lid and ring or aluminum foil. Place filled jars in oven with light on and allow to ripen to desired consistency. (I ripen mine 4 hours.) Place yogurt in refrigerator. Yogurt will keep in refrigerator for a good 4 weeks. Remember to save 1 cup of your homemade yogurt as a starter for your next batch.

*Do not use ultra-pasteurized milk or yogurt will not set.

**I sweeten my yogurt by adding ¾ cup organic fructose per 1 gallon of milk. You may choose to add more or less sweetener depending on your preferences. I add the fructose with the powdered milk.

LENTIL SKILLET DINNER (GF)

1 vegetable or chicken bouillon cube

1 cup lentils

1½ cups water

3 Tbsp. olive oil

2 tsp. minced garlic

1 large white onion, diced

1 cup mushrooms, sliced

2 yellow squash, sliced

2 zucchini squash, sliced

1 cup Roma tomatoes, chopped

1 cup fresh mozzarella, cubed

½ cup fresh basil, chopped

¼ cup fresh oregano, chopped

Spike® Seasoning to taste

In a medium-sized pot, combine bouillon cube, lentils, and water and cook until lentils are tender, about 10 minutes. While lentils are cooking, sauté garlic and onion in olive oil in a large skillet for 2 minutes over medium-high heat. Add mushrooms and squash and cook until tender. Toss lentils and cooked vegetables with remaining ingredients. If you are gluten intolerant, be sure to use a gluten-free bouillon.

VEGETABLE QUICHE

2 Tbsp. oil

1 tsp. garlic

¼ medium white onion, chopped

½ cup corn

½ green bell pepper, sliced

½ orange bell pepper, sliced

½ yellow bell pepper, sliced

¼ cup Anaheim pepper, chopped

1 cup spinach

2 eggs

⅓ cup milk

1 deep-dish pie shell

⅓ cup prepared quinoa

⅓ cup prepared wheat berries

⅓ cup prepared barley pearls

1 cup mozzarella cheese

1 Tbsp. basil, chopped

Preheat oven to 400°F. In a medium-sized skillet, sauté oil, garlic, onions, corn, and assorted peppers. When peppers are tender add spinach and cook until tender; this will only take a minute or two. In a separate bowl, combine quinoa, wheat berries, and barley pearls. Spoon grains and half of vegetable mixture into pie shell and sprinkle with half of cheese; repeat layers, ending with cheese. Top with basil. Whisk together eggs and milk and pour over basil. Bake for 30–45 minutes or until a knife inserted in the middle of quiche comes out clean. Complete your meal with a bowl of Homemade Tomato Soup.

WHOLE WHEAT BERRIES (WHOLE GRAIN WHEAT)

I use two methods to cook wheat berries.

5 cups water
2 cups wheat berries

In a medium sized pot with a tight-fitting lid, bring water and wheat berries to a rolling boil. Reduce heat to low and simmer for 1½ hours.
Or cook overnight in a slow cooker.

RED LENTIL SALAD (GF)

1 cup red lentils

1½ cups vegetable broth

1 cup diced Roma tomatoes

¾ cup diced green bell peppers

¾ cup red bell peppers

½ cup jicama root, cubed

½ cup pine nuts

¼ cup finely diced red onion

2 Tbsp. fresh chopped basil

2 Tbsp. fresh chopped Italian parsley

4 Tbsp. fresh chopped cilantro

2 Tbsp. fresh chopped mint

1 Tbsp. fresh chopped dill

Lemon wedges

Spike® seasoning to taste

Place lentils in broth and boil over medium heat until tender, 10–15 minutes. Drain lentils and cool. Prepare vegetables and herbs. Toss cooled lentils, vegetables, and herbs with lemon juice and Spike® seasoning as desired. If you are gluten intolerant, be sure to use a gluten-free bouillon.

BORSCHT (GF)

2 Tbsp. pickling spices

5 cups water

3 large beets, peeled and diced

2 large carrots, sliced

2 cups green cabbage, chopped

1 medium onion, chopped

2 tsp. minced garlic

6 Tbsp. vinegar

1 Tbsp. sugar

¼ tsp. black pepper

½ tsp. salt

Secure pickling spices in tea infuser or cheese cloth and place in a large stock pot. Add remaining ingredients and simmer over medium heat for 30 minutes or until beets are tender. Pluck out bag of pickling spices. Place 3 cups cooked vegetables in a blender or food processor and add soup liquid until smooth. Return puree to stock pot and combine with remaining vegetables and broth. Complete your meal with Russian cucumber salad.

RUSSIAN CUCUMBER SALAD (GF)

4 radishes, sliced

1 large cucumber, sliced

1 green onion, chopped

2 Tbsp. sour cream

Salt and pepper to taste

Combine all ingredients in medium-sized bowl and toss until vegetables are coated evenly.

ROASTED PORTABELLAS WITH SMOKED GOUDA
AND FENNEL (GF)

4 medium portabella mushrooms, washed and scored

3 Tbsp. olive oil

1 large fennel bulb, sliced

½ tsp. dried tarragon

Balsamic vinegar

1 cup grape tomatoes

4 ounces smoked Gouda cheese, shredded

½ cup fresh basil, chopped

¼ cup pine nuts

Salt to taste

Preheat oven to 350°F. Brush prepared mushroom caps with olive oil and place in baking dish, gill side down. Bake for 15 minutes. While mushrooms are baking, sauté fennel and tarragon in remaing olive oil in a small skillet. Remove from heat when fennel is tender and edges start browning. Remove mushrooms from oven and turn mushrooms so gill side is up. Brush mushrooms with balsamic vinegar. Add tomatoes and brush with more balsamic vinegar. Top with sautéed fennel and cheese. Return mushrooms to oven and bake for 10 minutes or until cheese has melted. Remove from oven and sprinkle with basil and pine nuts. Salt to taste.

CAULIFLOWER BAKE

1 head cauliflower

1 cup fresh or frozen peas

1 (15-oz.) can corn, drained

1 (5-oz.) can water chestnuts, chopped

¼ cup red bell pepper

Batter:

5 eggs

½ cup whole wheat flour

½ tsp. baking powder

2 Tbsp. sugar

1 pinch salt

1 cup milk

5 tsp. Dijon mustard

2 Tbsp. vinegar

2 Tbsp. olive oil

1 tsp. dried dill

½ tsp. turmeric

¼ tsp. onion powder

⅛ tsp. cayenne pepper

Garnish

½ cup feta crumbles

¼ cup fresh basil, chopped

½ cup fresh Roma tomatoes, chopped

Preheat oven to 450°F. In a large pot, cover cauliflower with water and boil until tender. Remove cauliflower from heat and drain. Place cauliflower in a greased 9 x 13 baking dish. Top with remaining vegetables.

Blend batter ingredients in a food processor until smooth. Gently pour batter over vegetables. Sprinkle garnish ingredients evenly over batter. Bake for 10 minutes. Reduce temperature to 350°F and bake for 20–25 minutes or until a knife inserted in the middle comes out clean. Allow to cool 5–10 minutes before serving.

EGGPLANT PARMESAN

1 spaghetti squash, baked

1 large eggplant peeled and cut into 1-inch slices

2 large eggs, whisked

2 cups, Italian seasoned bread crumbs

2 cups spaghetti sauce

¾ cup coarsely shredded Romano cheese

Oil

Preheat oven to 350°F. Run a fork back and forth along spaghetti squash flesh, scraping it out until it resembles spaghetti and place in a greased 9 x 13 baking dish. Dip eggplant slices in egg and coat with bread crumbs. Place coated eggplant on top of spaghetti squash. Place a dollop of spaghetti sauce on top of eggplant slice and sprinkle with Romano cheese. Bake at 350° for 30–45 minutes or until eggplant is tender.

CHEESE RAVIOLI WITH BUTTERNUT SQUASH SAUCE

1 package prepared cheese ravioli (found in freezer
   section at most grocery stores)

Butternut Squash Sauce (GF)

½ cup cooked butternut squash (frozen, canned, or
   fresh)

1 cup vegetable or chicken broth

2 cups milk

2 Tbsp. flour

2 Tbsp. butter

2 tsp. tarragon

¼ tsp. crushed garlic

Garnish:

1 medium tomato, chopped

¼ cup fresh basil, chopped

½ cup grated Romano cheese

Prepare ravioli according to package directions.
Place all sauce ingredients in blender and blend until
smooth. Transfer sauce to a large pot and cook 10 minutes over medium heat, stirring frequently. Ladle butternut
squash sauce over ravioli garnish and enjoy with a Spelt
and Barley Parmesan Bread Stick (see page 128). If you
are gluten intolerant, be sure to use gluten-free broth.

CHEESE RAVIOLI WITH TOMATO BASIL SAUCE

1 package prepared cheese ravioli (found in freezer
     section at most grocery stores)

Tomato Basil Sauce (GF)

   2 tsp. garlic, crushed

   2 Tbsp. olive oil

   8 Roma tomatoes, chopped

   1 cup cream

   ½ tsp. salt or ½ tsp. chicken bouillon granules

   ½ cup Parmesan cheese

   1 cup fresh basil

Prepare ravioli according to package directions.
In a medium saucepan, sauté garlic in olive oil. Add
tomatoes and cream. When cream starts bubbling, add
salt or chicken bouillon granules and Parmesan cheese.
Mix in basil and ladle over cheese ravioli. Enjoy with a
Spelt Barley Parmesan Bread Stick (see page 128). If you
are gluten intolerant, be sure to use gluten-free bouillon.

PUMPKIN SOUP (GF)

1 4-pound pie pumpkin or 4 cups canned or frozen
  pumpkin

2 cups vegetable or chicken broth

2 cups milk

¼ tsp. ginger

¼ tsp. cinnamon

¼ tsp. nutmeg

2 tsp. tarragon

Preheat oven to 350°F. Cut pumpkin in half and scrape clean. Place upside down on a cookie sheet lined with aluminum foil and bake for 45 minutes. Scoop pumpkin flesh from outer shell and place in blender. Blend pumpkin with remaining ingredients until smooth. Heat to desired temperature and serve. If you are gluten intolerant, be sure to use a gluten-free bouillon.

TOMATO SOUP (GF)

2 quarts tomatoes

1 medium onion, chopped

1 stalk celery, chopped

4 sprigs fresh parsley

2 Tbsp. sugar

1 tsp. salt

½ tsp. black pepper

Place tomatoes in hot water until skins split. Immediately place in cold water and skins will slip off. Place all ingredients in a large stock pot over medium high-heat, stirring frequently. Cook until all vegetables are tender. Carefully spoon soup into a food processor and blend until smooth. Serve, bottle, or refrigerate for future use.

STIR FRIED RICE (GF)

2 Tbsp. oil

1 tsp. garlic

½ medium onion, chopped

1 celery stalk, chopped

1 cup bok choy, chopped

½ cup mushrooms, sliced

1 cup pea pods

½ cup frozen peas and carrots, thawed

2 cups cooked rice

1 Tbsp. soy sauce (we like Golden Mountain®
    Seasoning Sauce)

¼ tsp. salt

1 Tbsp. sesame seeds

Place oil, garlic, and all vegetables in skillet, reserving pea pods and peas and carrots. Cook over medium-high heat, stirring frequently. When vegetables are tender, add pea pods and peas and carrots, rice, seasoning sauce, and salt. When heated thoroughly after 2–3 minutes, sprinkle with sesame seeds and serve. If you are gluten intolerant, be sure to use gluten-free soy sauce.

JAMAICAN TOFU OVER RICE (GF)

1 cup water

1 cup rice

2 Tbsp. safflower oil

1 tsp. minced garlic

1 medium onion, chopped

1 tsp. curry powder

1 tsp. thyme

½ tsp. allspice

½ tsp. crushed red pepper flakes

½ tsp. black pepper

½ lime, juiced

½ cup chopped cilantro

1 (15-oz.) can black beans, drained and rinsed

2 cups diced Roma tomatoes

1 (20-oz.) can pineapple chunks

1 (14-oz.) package firm tofu, cubed

In a heavy-bottomed saucepan with a tight-fitting lid, boil and rice over high heat for 15 minutes. Remove from heat and set aside for 10 minutes and then fluff. Do not lift lid and peek at rice while it is resting. If you have a rice cooker, just add water and rice, press the lever, and fluff rice when lever pops up. In large saucepan, combine oil, garlic, and onions. Cook until tender. Add remaining ingredients except tofu. Simmer over medium heat for 10 minutes. Stir in tofu and spoon mixture over rice.

SPICY CARIBBEAN RICE (GF)

5 cups water

2 cups rice

1 medium onion, chopped

2 tsp. minced garlic

1 bell pepper, chopped

1 stalk celery, chopped

2 Tbsp. safflower oil

½ tsp. black pepper

1 tsp. thyme

1 tsp. curry powder

4 Tbsp. brown sugar

4 sprigs fresh parsley

2 vegetable bouillon cubes

1 (15-oz.) can black-eyed peas, drained

1 (15-oz.) can garbanzo beans, drained

In a heavy-bottomed saucepan with a tight-fitting lid, boil 3 cups water and 2 cups rice over high heat for 15 minutes. Remove from heat, set aside for 10 minutes, and then fluff. Do not lift lid and peek at rice while it is resting. If you have a rice cooker, just add water and rice and press the lever. Fluff rice when lever pops up.

In a medium saucepan, cook onion, garlic, bell pepper, and celery in oil until tender. Add spices, bouillon cubes, and remaining 2 cups of water and cook 10 minutes uncovered. Add black-eyed peas and garbanzo beans and heat thoroughly. To serve, pour black-eyed pea mixture over rice. If you are gluten intolerant, be sure to use a gluten-free bouillon.

SUMMER DELIGHT SALAD (GF)

2 grapefruits, sectioned and cut into 1-inch pieces

Fruit of one pomegranate

1 cup strawberries, sliced

1 cup blueberries

1 cup raspberries

Juice of 1 lime

Mint leaves for garnish

Place washed and prepared fruit in a medium bowl. Drizzle lime juice over fruit and gently toss. Garnish with mint leaves.

CHIPOTLE PUMPKIN SOUP (GF)

1 cup pumpkin puree

⅔ cup Chipotle Sauce (see recipe on page 136)

1½ cups vegetable bouillon

1 cup Roma tomatoes, chopped

½ cup cilantro, chopped

1 avocado, cubed

½ cup manchego cheese, grated

Blue corn tortilla chips

Place pumpkin, chipotle sauce, and bouillon in a medium-sized pot and simmer for 10 minutes. Stir in tomatoes and ladle into bowls. Garnish soup with cilantro, avocado, and cheese. Serve with blue corn tortilla chips. If you are gluten intolerant, be sure to use a gluten-free bouillon.

EGGS IN THE FIELD (GF)

½ cup water

2 bunches fresh spinach

Olive oil

4 eggs

3 Tbsp. cream

¼ tsp. nutmeg

Salt to taste

Hollandaise sauce, optional

Preheat oven to 350°F. In a medium-sized pot, bring water to boil and add spinach. When spinach turns brilliant green, quickly transfer to colander and drain thoroughly. Oil a 9 x 9 baking dish and add spinach. Make 4 depressions large enough to hold an egg. Crack a raw egg over each depression. Drizzle cream over spinach. Sprinkle nutmeg over spinach and eggs. Bake for 18–20 minutes. For a special occasion (any time you have an excuse to enjoy high-fat foods, like on Mother's Day), I top the baked eggs with hollandaise sauce before serving.

HOLLANDAISE SAUCE

½ cup melted butter

4 egg yolks*

½ cup cream

2 Tbsp. lemon juice

1 tsp. Dijon mustard

½ tsp. nutmeg

In a small saucepan, whisk melted butter and egg yolks. Add cream and lemon juice to egg mixture and cook over medium-low heat, stirring continuously until sauce begins to thicken. Remove sauce from heat and stir in mustard and nutmeg.

***Raw eggs have been found to contain Salmonella bacteria.** The Centers for Disease Control and Prevention estimate that 1 in 10,000 eggs in America contain Salmonella. I therefore advise anyone who would like to eliminate the risk of Salmonella infection to use pasteurized eggs. Pasteurized eggs are commonly found in the refrigerated section of your local grocery store. People in high-risk groups such as the elderly, children, pregnant women, and those with a weakened immune system should always use pasteurized eggs when making recipes that call for raw eggs or if you are planning on eating raw cookie dough.

EGGPLANT CACCIATORE (GF)

6 cups water

1 (12-oz.) package whole wheat fettuccine pasta OR
    gluten-free pasta

1 large eggplant, cubed

2 tsp. minced garlic

1 medium onion, chopped

2 Tbsp olive oil

2 (14.5-oz.) cans diced Italian tomatoes

2 (8-oz.) cans tomato sauce

½ cup Concord grape juice

¼ tsp. black pepper

½ tsp. whole celery seed

1½ tsp. dried oregano

3 bay leaves

½ cup Parmesan cheese

In a large pot, bring water to boil. Add pasta and cook 6–7 minutes or to desired tenderness. Remove from heat and drain. In a large saucepan, sauté eggplant, garlic, and onion in olive oil until onions turn translucent. Add remaining ingredients, except Parmesan cheese, and simmer over medium heat for 20 minutes or until eggplant is tender. To serve, place pasta on plate and top with eggplant cacciatore sauce. Sprinkle with Parmesan cheese. Complete your meal with a green salad and a slice of French bread.

VEGETABLES WITH THAI SWEET CHILI SAUCE AND RICE (GF)

3 Tbsp. peanut oil

2 Tbsp. garlic, minced

1 medium onion, chopped

2 large carrots, thinly sliced

1½ cup broccoli flowerets

2 stalks of celery, sliced

1½ cup bean sprouts

1 (15-oz.) can baby corn, drained

1 (5-oz.) can bamboo shoots

1 (5-oz.) can sliced water chestnuts

Thai sweet chili sauce to taste (we prefer the Mae Ploy® brand)

Heat peanut oil in wok and add garlic and onions. Next add carrots, broccoli, celery, bean sprouts, and canned vegetables. Do not overcook. Pour sweet chili sauce onto vegetables and toss. Serve over rice. I serve this in bowls so that the yummy sauce also covers the rice.

SESAME BABY BOK CHOY (GF)

3 Tbsp. peanut oil

1½ tsp. garlic, crushed

4 baby bok choy, washed and chopped, if desired

4 Tbsp. sesame seeds

Seasoning sauce or soy sauce to taste

Salt to taste

Heat oil in wok or skillet on high heat. Add garlic to oil followed by prepared bok choy. When bok choy turns a brighter shade of green and becomes tender, remove from heat. Stir in sesame seeds, seasoning sauce, and salt to taste. I use about 3–5 teaspoons seasoning sauce and ½ teaspoon salt. If you are gluten intolerant, be sure to use gluten-free soy sauce.

SPRING ROLLS (GF)

1 cup bean sprouts

1 stalk celery, finely sliced

½ cup matchstick carrots

½ cup green onion, finely chopped

½ cup mushrooms, minced

1 cup Napa cabbage, grated

2 avocados, cubed

½ pound tiny pre-cooked salad shrimp, optional

Warm water

1 package rice spring roll wrappers

Peanut sauce

Plum sauce

Prepare vegetables and toss with shrimp (if desired) in a large bowl. Place 1 cup warm water in a shallow and wide pot or bowl. Place one wrapper in water and allow to rest until soft and pliable, 20–30 seconds. If wrapper gets too soft, decrease length of time in water. Place softened wrapper on a large plate. Place ¼ cup filling in middle of wrapper and fold filled wrapper like a burrito or egg roll. In other words, fold ends and then roll closed. Serve with peanut sauce and plum sauce.

GREEN CHILE ENCHILADAS (GF)

6–8 corn tortillas

Enchilada Filling:
- 3 Tbsp. oil
- 2 cups cooked rice
- 1 yellow squash, sliced
- 1 onion, chopped
- 1 zucchini, sliced
- 1 cup corn
- 1 cup black beans
- 1 cup kidney beans
- 1 tsp. cumin

Green Chile Sauce:
- ¼ cup butter
- 1 tsp. garlic
- 1 medium onion, finely chopped
- 2 cups milk
- 3 Tbsp. flour
- 1 tsp. vegetable or chicken bouillon granules
- ¼ tsp. salt
- 1 tsp. cumin
- 1 tsp. coriander
- 1 can diced green chiles
- 1 cup grated Monterey Jack cheese

Garnish:
- Fresh chopped cilantro
- Roma tomatoes, chopped
- Avocado, sliced

Preheat oven to 350°F. Heat oil in saucepan over medium heat and cook onion and squash until tender. In a large bowl, mix all filling ingredients, including cooked onion and squash. In a saucepan, melt butter and then add garlic and onion and cook until onion is translucent. Remove pan from burner and stir in flour until a paste forms. Return to burner and drizzle in milk, stirring continuously until mixture thickens. When all the milk has been incorporated, add bouillon granules, salt, cumin, coriander, and green chiles.

Grease a 9 x 13 baking pan, place ½–¾ cup of filling in tortilla and roll up. Place tortilla in prepared baking dish, seam side down. Once baking dish is filled with stuffed tortillas, cover with green chile sauce and Monterey Jack cheese. Bake for 20–25 minutes. Cool for 5 minutes and garnish as desired. If you are gluten intolerant, be sure to use a gluten-free bouillon.

DAHL SOUP (GF)

4 cups water

4 vegetable bouillon cubes

2 cups red lentils

1 tsp. minced garlic

1 medium onion, chopped

½ tsp. turmeric

1 Tbsp. garam masala

¼ tsp. cayenne pepper

1 tsp. ground cumin

1 Tbsp. granulated white sugar

2 cups diced Roma tomatoes

1 (13.5-oz.) can coconut milk

½ cup chopped cilantro

In a large saucepan over medium heat, combine all ingredients except tomatoes, coconut milk, and cilantro. When lentils and onions are tender, add tomatoes, coconut milk, and cilantro. Serve hot. If you are gluten intolerant, be sure to use a gluten-free bouillon.

QUINOA SALAD (GF)

2 cups cooked quinoa

1 cup grape tomatoes

1 cup raw fennel, thinly sliced

1 cup cashews

¾ cup mint, chopped

⅓ cup green onions, chopped

½ cup red bell pepper, diced

½ cup dates, seeded and chopped

6 Tbsp. feta cheese crumbles

Place prepared ingredients in medium bowl, add Honey Tarragon Dressing (see recipe below), and toss.

HONEY TARRAGON DRESSING (GF)

¼ cup olive oil

2 Tbsp. lemon juice

2 Tbsp. honey

1 Tbsp. dried tarragon

¼ tsp. salt

Place all ingredients in food processor and blend until smooth.

FIVE "P" SOUP (GF)

5 cups vegetable broth

2 tsp. coriander, ground

¼ tsp. black pepper

1 large potato, cubed

3 parsnips, sliced

2 cups pumpkin, cubed

1 stalk celery

1 onion, diced

2 tsp. garlic

1 cup fresh or frozen peas

½ cup fresh parsley, chopped

In a large pot, combine broth, spices, potato, parsnip pumpkin, celery, onion, and garlic. When vegetables are tender, add peas and parsley. Cook only until peas are warmed through. If you are gluten intolerant, be sure to use a gluten-free broth.

LEMON ASPARAGUS SOUP

1 pound asparagus cut into 1-inch pieces

3 Tbsp. butter

1 medium onion, chopped

¼ tsp. crushed garlic

¼ cup flour

⅓ cup freshly squeezed lemon juice

1 tsp. ground coriander seed

½ tsp. ground thyme

¼ tsp. ground allspice

2 cups milk

4 cups vegetable broth

½ cup chopped watercress

In a medium pot, place prepared asparagus in broth and boil until tender. In a large skillet, sauté butter, onions, and garlic until onions are tender. Remove from heat and stir in flour. Once flour, garlic, and onions have formed a paste, add broth from asparagus, lemon juice, and spices. Return pot to burner and stir until mixture is the consistency of gravy. Pour mixture and milk into a food processor and blend until smooth. Reserving 1 cup of cooked asparagus, add remaining asparagus to food processor and blend until smooth. Add watercress and simmer for 5 minutes. Add reserved asparagus to soup before serving.

EZEKIEL BREAD MUFFINS

"That which doesn't kill you will make you stronger." I believe Ezekiel said this after living on Ezekiel bread for two years! Just kidding!

In the Holy Bible, Ezekiel 4:9 gives a rough recipe for what is known as Ezekiel bread. When I examined the flours, I came to the belief that God was giving Ezekiel a recipe which would make a plant-based complete protein bread. The bread is dense and holds together better as a muffin than a sliced loaf.

¾ cup whole wheat flour

¾ cup spelt flour

¼ cup millet flour

¼ cup lentils

¼ cup barley

2 Tbsp. pinto bean flour

2 Tbsp. red kidney bean flour

1 tsp. salt

2 tsp. baking powder

2 tsp. oil

5 Tbsp. honey

1–1½ cups water, depending on texture of flours

Vegetable shortening for muffin cups or muffin cup liners

Preheat oven to 375°F. In a large bowl, mix all dry ingredients together, followed by liquids. Stir only until just mixed. Grease muffin cups or use muffin cup liners. Spoon batter into prepared muffin cups and bake for 20–25 minutes or until a toothpick inserted comes out clean.

CAMOUFLAGED EZEKIEL BREAD MUFFINS

I thought the Ezekiel bread was fine for what it was; however, the children weren't thrilled with the muffins, so I went to work in the kitchen, added a few ingredients and voila! They were gobbled up in a blink! I mean, who wouldn't? Basically I converted a dense muffin into a light, moist, carrot cake muffin without altering the flours.

    2 Tbsp. pinto beans
    2 Tbsp. red kidney bean
    ¾ cup whole wheat flour
    ¾ cup spelt flour
    ¼ cup millet flour
    ¼ cup barley flour
    ¼ cup lentils
    1 teaspoon salt
    ¾ tsp. baking soda
    1½ tsp. baking powder
    1½ tsp. cinnamon
    1 cup buttermilk
    2 eggs
    ¼ cup honey
    1 cup applesauce
    1 cup shredded carrots
    1 cup raisins
    Vegetable shortening for muffin cups or muffin cup liners

Grind beans and other whole grains or berries into flour using food processor or mill. Preheat oven to 375°F. In a large bowl, mix all dry ingredients, followed by liquids and finally applesauce, carrots, and raisins. Grease muffin cups. Spoon batter into prepared muffin cups and bake for 20–25 minutes or when a toothpick inserted into the middle comes out clean.

ROSEMARY VEGETABLE BAKE (GF)

4 medium turnips, cubed

4 large carrots, sliced

4 large parsnips, sliced

Olive oil

4 Tbsp. melted butter

4 Tbsp. orange juice concentrate

1 tsp. cinnamon

½ tsp. ginger

Topping

1 medium onion, diced

2 Tbsp. butter

2 Tbsp. olive oil

8 ounces fresh sliced mushrooms

Salt

1 Tbsp. fresh chopped rosemary

Preheat oven to 350°F. Wash and prepare vegetables. Oil bottom and sides of a 9 x 13 baking dish. Place prepared vegetables in bottom of baking dish. In a small bowl whisk melted butter, orange juice concentrate, cinnamon, and ginger. Drizzle over vegetables. Bake uncovered for 40 minutes.

While vegetables are cooking, prepare topping. In a large skillet over medium heat, cook onions in butter and olive oil. When onions are tender, add mushrooms. Cook until onions and mushrooms are caramelized. Salt to taste. When vegetable have finished baking, top with onions, mushrooms, and fresh rosemary. If the children are not going to be home for dinner, I add blue cheese crumbles for extra zing!

CREAMY POTATO CORN SOUP (GF)

5 cups vegetable or chicken broth

1 medium onion, chopped

2 medium potatoes, cubed

2 cups fresh or frozen corn

1 teaspoon minced garlic

½ cup prepared red lentils

½ cup fresh spinach

Garnish

2 tablespoons of each: chopped red, yellow, and green
   bell peppers

¼ cup chopped Roma tomatoes

⅛ teaspoon white pepper

In a large pot combine broth, potatoes, garlic, and onion.
When potatoes are tender, add corn. Puree vegetables
in blender until smooth. Return pureed mixture to pot and
add lentils. Simmer until lentils are hot. Stir in spinach and
cook until spinach turns brilliant green. Garnish and serve.
If you are gluten intolerant, be sure to use a gluten-free
bouillon.

APPENDIX B:

RECIPE INDEX

RECIPE INDEX

APPENDIX C:

SUGGESTED READINGS AND RESOURCES

COMPARATIVE STUDIES OF RELIGIOUS DIETARY GUIDELINES:

Ahmadani, M. Y., M. Riaz, A. Fawwad, M. Z. Hydrie, R. Hakeem, A. Basi. "Glycaemic Trend Furing Ramadan in Fasting Diabetic Subjects: A Study from Pakistan."*Pakistan Journal of Biological Sciences* 11, no. 16 (2008): 2044–47.

Akhan, G., S. Kutluhan, H. R. Koyuncuoglu. "Is There Any Change of Stroke Incidence During Ramadan?" *Acta Neurologica Scandinavia* 101, no. 4 (2000): 259–61.

Aksungar, Fehime B., Aynur E. Topkaya, and Mahmut Akyildiz. "Interleukin-6, C-Reactive Protein and Biochemical Parameters During Prolonged Intermittent Fasting." *Annals of Nutrition & Motabolism* 51, no. 1 (Mar. 2007): 88–95.

Al-Khawari, Mona, Ahlam Al-Ruwayeh, Khaled Al-Doub, and Jeremy Allgrove. "Adolescents on Basal-bolus Insulin Can Fast During Ramadan." *Pediatric Diabetes* 11 (2010): 96–100. doi:10.1111lj.1399–5448.2009.00544.x

Al Suwaidi, J., A. Bener, H. A. Hajar, and M.T. Numan. "Does Hospitalization for Congestive Heart Failure Occur More Frequently in Ramadan: A Population-based Study (1991–2001)." *International Journal of Cardiology* 96, no. 2 (2004): 217–21.

Alexander, Heather, Laura P. Lockwood, Mary A. Harris, and Christopher L. Melby. "Risk Factors for Cardiovascular Disease and Diabetes in Two Groups of Hispanic Americans with Differing Dietary Habits." *Journal of the American College of Nutrition* 18, no. 2 (1999): 127–36.

Armstrong, Bruce, Helen Clarke, Craig Martin, William Ward, Neroli Norman, and John Masarei. "Urinary Sodium and Blood Pressure in Vegetarians." *The American Journal of Clnical Nutrition* 32, no. 12 (1979): 2472–76.

Beilin, Lawrence J., Ian L Rouse, Bruce K Armstrong, Barrie M Margetts, and Robert Vandongen. "Vegetarian Diet and Blood Pressure Levels: Incidental or Causal Association?" *The American Journal of Clinical Nutrition* 48 (1988): 806–10.

Bener, A, B. Colakoglu, H. Mobayed, A. El Hakeem, A. A. Al

Mulla, and A. Sabbah. "Does Hospitalization for Asthma and Allergic Diseases Occur More Frequently in Ramadan Fasting: A Population-based Study (2000–2004)." *European Annals of Allergy and Clinical Immunology* 38, no. 4 (2006): 109–12.

Brathwaite, N., H.S. Fraser, N. Modeste, H. Broome, R. King, L. M. Butler, A. H. Wu, R. Wang, W. P. Koh, J. M. Yuan, and M. C. Yu. "A Vegetable-Fruit-Soy Dietary Pattern Protects Against Breast Cancer Among Postmenopausal Singapore Chinese Women." *The American Journal of Clinical Nutrition* 13, no. 1 (2010): 34–9.

Centers for Disease Control. "Angiostrongylus Infection Fact Sheet." Division of Parasitic Infection. Last reviewed September 18, 2008, http://www.cdc.gov/ncidod/dpd/parasites/angiostrongylus/factsht_angiostrongylus.htm#howinfected

Chamsi-Pasha, H., and W. H. AhmedWH. "The Effect of Fasting in Ramadan on Patients with Heart Disease." *Saudi Medical Journal* 25, no. 1(2004): 47–51.

Chanarin, I., V. Malkowska, A. M. O'Hea, M. G. Rinsler, and A. B. Price. "Megaloblastic Anaemia in a Vegetarian Hindu Community." *Lancet* 2, no. 8,465 (1985): 1168–72.

Chanarin, I. and E. Stephenson. "Vegetarian Diet and Cobalamin Deficiency: Their Association with Tuberculosis." *Journal of Clinical Pathology* 41, no. 7 (1988): 759–62.

Chaouachi Anis, John B. Leiper, Nizar Souissi, Aaron J. Coutts, and Karim Chamari. "Effects of Ramadan Intermittent Fasting on Sports Performance and Training: A Review." *International Journal of Sports Physiology and Performance* 4, no. 4. (2009): 419–34.

Chen, C-W., Y-L Lin, T-K Lin, C-T Lin, B-C Chen, and C-L Lin. "Total Cardiovascular Risk Profile of Taiwanese Vegetarians." *European Journal of Clinical Nutrition* 62, no. 1 (2008): 138–44.

Chennaoui, Mounir, François Desgorces, Catherine Drogou, Bechir Boudjemaa, Armand Tomaszewski, Frédéric Depiesse, Pascal Burnat, Hakim Chalabi, and Danielle Gomez-Merino. "Effects of Ramadan Fasting on Physical

Performance and Metabolic, Hormonal, and Inflammatory Parameters in Middle-distance Runners." *Applied Physiology, Nutrition, and Motabolism* 34, no. 4. (2009): 587–94.

Choi, Dongil, Jae Hoon Lim, Dong-Chull Choi, Seung Woon Paik, Sun-Hee Kim, and Sun Huh. "Toxocariasis and Ingestion of Raw Cow Liver in Patients with Eosinophilia." *Korean Journal of Parisitology* 46, no. 3 (2008): 139–43. doi: 10.3347.kjp.2008.46.3.139.

Cohen A. "Seasonal Daily Effect on the Number of Births in Israel." *Journal of the Royal Statistical Society, Series C (Applied Statistics)* 32, no. 3 (1983): 228–35.

Craig, W. J. and A. R. Mangels; "American Dietetic Association Position of the American Dietetic Association: Vegetarian Diets." *Journal of American Dietetic Association* 109, no. 7 (2009): 1266–82.

Cross, J. H., J. Eminson, and B. A. Wharton. "Ramadan and Birth Weight at Full Term in Asian Moslem Pregnant Women in Birmingham." *Archives of Disease in Childhood* 65, no. 10 (1990): 1053–56.

Cui, Xiaohui, Qi Dai, Marilyn Tseng, Xiao-Ou Shu, Yu-Tang Gao, and Wei Zheng. "Dietary Patterns and Breast Cancer Risk in the Shanghai Breast Cancer Study." *Cancer Epidemiology, Biomarkers, & Prevention* 16, no. 7 (2007): 1443–8.

Díaz Camacho, Sylvia Paz, Kaethe Willms, Ma. del Carmen de la Cruz Otero, Magda Luz Zazueta Ramos, Sergio Bayliss Gaxiola, Rafael Castro Velázquez, Ignacio Osuna Ramírez, Angel Bojórquez Contreras, Edith Hilario Torres Montoya, and Sergio Gonzáles. "Acute Outbreak of Gnathostomiasis in a Fishing Community in Sinaloa, Mexico." *Parasitology International* 52, no. 2 (2003): 133–40.

Dikensoy, E., O. Balat, B. Cebesoy, A. Ozkur, H. Cicek, and G. Can. "Effect of Fasting During Ramadan on Fetal Development and Maternal Health." *Journal of Obstetrics and Gynaecol Research* 34, no. 4 (2008): 494–98.

Dikensoy, E., O. Balat, B. Cebesoy, A. Ozkur, H. Cicek, and G. Can. "The Effect of Ramadan Fasting on Maternal

Serum Lipids, Cortisol Levels, and Fetal Development." *Archives of Gynecology and Obstetrics* 279, no. 2 (2009): 119–23.

Dos Santos Silva, Isabel, Punam Mangtani, Valerie McCormack, Dee Bhakta, Leena Sevak, and Anthony J. McMichael AJ. "Lifelong Vegetarianism and Risk of Breast Cancer: A Population-based Case-control Study Among South Asian Migrant Women Living in England." *International Journal of Cancer* 99, no. 2 (2002): 238–44.

Drescher, Michael J., E. A. Alpert, T. Zalut, R. Torgovicky, and Z. Wimpfheimer. "Prophylactic Etoricoxib Is Effective in Preventing Yom Kippur Headache: A Placebo-Controlled Double-Blind and Randomized Trial of Prophylaxis for Ritual Fasting Headache." *Headache: The Journal of Head and Face Pain* 50, no. 8 (2010): 1328–1334.

Drescher, Michael J. and Yonatan Elstein. "Prophylactic COX 2 Inhibitor: An End to the Yom Kippur Headache." *Headache: The Journal of Head and Face Pain* 46, no. 10 (2006): 1487–91.

Enstrom, James E. and Leseter Breslow. "Lifestyle and Reduced Mortality among Active California Mormons, 1980–2004." *Preventive Medicine* 46, no. 2 (2008): 133–136.

Enstrom, James E. "Health Practices and Cancer Mortality Among Active California Mormons." *Journal of the National Cancer Institute* 81, no. 23 (1989): 1807–14.

Fønnebø, V. "Mortality in Norwegian Seventh-Day Adventists 1962–1986." *Journal of Clinical Epidemiology* 45, no. 2 (1992): 157–67.

Franco, Manuel, Ana V. Diez Roux, Thomas A. Glass, Benjamin Caballero, and Frederick L. Brancati. "Neighborhood Characteristics and Availability of Healthy Foods in Baltimore." *American Journal of Preventative Medicine* 35, no. 6 (2008): 561–7.

Fraser, G. E., W. L. Beeson, and R. L. Phillips. "Diet and Lung Cancer in California Seventh-day Adventists." *American Journal of Epidemiology* 133, no. 7 (1991): 683–93.

Fraser, Gary E., Joan Sabaté, W. Lawrence Beeson, and T.

Martin Strahan. "A Possible Protective Effect of Nut Consumption on Risk of Coronary Heart Disease: The Adventist Health Study." *Archives of Internal Medicine* 152, no 7.
(1992): 1416–24.

Fraser, Gary E. and David J. Shavlik. "Risk Factors for All-
cause and Coronary Heart Disease Mortality in the Oldest-
old: The Adventist Health Study." *Archives of Internal
Medicine* 157, no. 19 (1997): 2249–58.

Fraser, Gary E. "Associations Between Diet and Cancer, Ischemic Heart Disease, and All-cause Mortality in Non-His-
panic White California Seventh-day Adventists." *American
Journal of Clinical Nutrition* 70, Supplement (1997):
532S–538S.

Fu, Chin-Hua, Cheryl C. H. Yang, Chin-Lon Lin, and Terry
B. J. Kuo. "Effects of Long-term Vegetarian Diets on Cardiovascular Autonomic Functions in Healthy Postmenopausal Women." *American Journal of Cardiology* 97, no. 3
(2006): 380–3.

Grundmann, E. "Cancer Morbidity and Mortality in USA
Mormons and Seventh-day Adventists." *Archives d Anato-
mie et de Cytologie Pathologiques* 40, no. 2 (1992): 73–78.

Haq, S.M. and H. H. Dayal. "Chronic Liver Disease and
Consumption of Raw Oysters: A Potentially Lethal Combination—A Review of Vibrio Vulnificus Septicemia."
American Journal of Gastroenterology 100, no. 5 (2005):
1195–9.

He, Yuna, Guansheng Ma, Fengying Zhai, Yanping Li, Yisong
Hu, Edith J. M. Feskens, and Xiaoguang Yang. "Dietary
Patterns and Glucose Tolerance Abnormalities in Chinese
Adults." *Diabetes Care* 32, no. 11 (2009): 1972–6.

Herman, Joanna S. and Peter L. Chiodini. "Gnathostomiasis,
Another Emerging Imported Disease." *Clinical Microbiol-
ogy Reviews* 22, no. 3 (2009): 484–92.

Hirayama T. "Mortality in Japanese With Life-styles Similar
to Seventh-Day Adventists: Strategy for Risk Reduction by
Life-style Modification." *National Cancer Institute Mono-
graphs* 69 (1985): 143–53.

Horne, Benjamin D., Heidi T. May, Jeffrey L. Anderson, Abdallah G. Kfoury, Beau M. Bailey, Brian S. McClure, Dale G. Renlund, Donald L. Lappé, John F. Carlquist, Patrick W. Fisher, Robert R. Pearson, Tami L. Bair, TEd D. Adams, and Joseph B. Muhlestein. "Usefulness of Routine Periodic Fasting to Lower Risk of Coronary Artery Disease in Patients Undergoing Coronary Angiography." *American Journal of Cardiology* 102, no. 7 (2008): 814–819.

Hung, Chien-Jung, Po-Chao Huang, Yi-Hwei Li, Shao-Chun Lu, Low-Tone Ho, and Hsu-Fang Chou. "Taiwanese Vegetarians Have Higher Insulin Sensitivity than Omnivores." *British Journal of Nutrition* 95, no. 1 (2006): 129–35.

Kaplan, Michael, Arthur I. Eidelman, and Yeshaya Aboulafia. "Fasting and the Precipitation of Labor: The Yom Kippur Effect." *JAMA* 250, no. 10 (1983): 1317–8.

Katibi, I. A., A. A. Akande, B. J. Bojuwoye, and A. B. Okesina. "Blood Sugar Control Among Fasting Muslims with Type 2 Diabetes Mellitus in Ilorin." *Nigerian Journal of Medicine* 10, no. 3 (2001): 132–4.

Kavehmanesh, Zohreh and Hassan Abolghasemi. "Maternal Ramadan Fasting and Neonatal Health." *Journal of Perinatology* 24, no. 12 (2004): 748–50.

Kennedy, Erin D., Rebecca L. Hall, Susan P. Montgomery, David G. Pyburn, and Jeffrey L. Jones "Trichinellosis Surveillance—United States, 2002–2007." *Centers for Disease Control and Prevention. MMWR Surveillance Summit* 58, no. 9 (2009): 1–7.

Kirkendall, D. T., J. B. Leiper, Z. Bartagi, J. Dvorak, and Y. Zerguini. "The Influence of Ramadan on Physical Performance Measures in Young Muslim Footballers." *Journal of Sports Science* 26, no. 3 supplement (2008): S15-27.

Larson, Nicole I., Mary T. Story, and Melissa C. Nelson. "Neighborhood Environments: Disparities in Access to Healthy Foods in the U.S." *American Journal of Preventative Medicine* 36, no. 1 (2009): 74–81.

Leung, F. W. "Etiologic Factors of Chronic Constipation—

Review of the Scientific Evidence." *Digestive Diseases and Sciences* 52 (2007): 313–316.

Lurie, S., C. Baider, M. Boaz, V. Sulema, A. Golan, and O Sadan. "Fasting Does Not Precipitate Onset of Labour." *Journal of Obstetrics and Gynaecology* 30, no. 1 (2010): 35–7.

Meckel, Y., A. Ismaeel, A. Eliakim. "The Effect of the Ramadan Fast on Physical Performance and Dietary Habits in Adolescent Soccer Players." *European Journal of Applied Physiology* 102, no. 6 (2008): 651–7.

Melby, Christopher L., David G. Goldflies, Gerald C. Hyner, and Roseann M. Lyle. "Relation Between Vegetarian/Nonvegetarian Diets and Blood Pressure in Black and White Adults." *American Journal of Public Health* 79, no. 9 (1989): 1283–88.

Merrill, Ray M. and Jeffrey A. Folsom. "Female Breast Cancer Incidence and Survival in Utah According to Religious Preference, 1985–1999." *BMC Cancer* 5 no. 49 (2005).

Merrill, Ray M. and Joseph L. Lyon. "Cancer Incidence among Mormons and Non-Mormons in Utah (United States) 1995–1999." *Preventive Medicine* 40, no. 5 (2005): 535–541.

Mills, P. K., W. L. Beeson, D. E. Abbey, G. E. Fraser, and R. L. Phillips. "Dietary Habits and Past Medical History as Related to Fatal Pancreas Cancer Risk Among Adventists." *Cancer* 61, no. 12 (1988): 2578–85.

Mills, P. K., W. L. Beeson, D. E. Abbey, and G. E. Fraser. "Bladder Cancer in a Low Risk Population: Results from the Adventist Health Study." *American Journal of Epidemiology* 133, no. 3 (1991): 230–39.

Mills, P. K., W. L. Beeson, D. E. Abbey, and G. E. Fraser. Cancer Incidence among California Seventh-Day Adventists, 1976–1982." *American Journal of Clinical Nutrition* 59, no. 5 supplement (1994): 1136S-1142S.

Mosek, A. and A. D. Korczyn. "Yom Kippur Headache." *Neurology* 45, no. 11 (1995): 1953–5.

Muller-Lissner, S.A., M. A. Kamm, C. Scarppignato, and A. Wald. "Myths and Misconceptions about Chronic Constipation." *American Journal of Gastroenterology* 100, no. 1

(2005): 232–242.

National Institutes of Health http://www.nih.gov/

Nettleton, Jennifer A., Joseph F. Polak, Russell Tracy, Gregory L Burke, and David R. Jacobs Jr. "Dietary Patterns and Incident Cardiovascular Disease in the Multi-Ethnic Study of Atherosclerosis." *American Journal of Clinical Nutrition* 90, no. 3 (2009): 647–54.

"Obesity, Diabetes, Hypertension, and Vegetarian Status Among Seventh-Day Adventists in Barbados: Preliminary Results." *Ethnicity and Disease* 13, no. 1 (2003): 34–9.

Office of Dietary Supplements website http://dietary-supplements.info.nih.gov/index.aspx

"Outbreak of Vibrio Parahaemolyticus Infections Associated with Eating Raw Oysters—Pacific Northwest, 1997" Centers for Disease Control http://www.cdc.gov/mmwr/preview/mmwrhtml/00053377.htm

Pawlak, R. and M. Sovyanhadi. "Prevalence of Overweight and Obesity among Seventh-day Adventist African American and Caucasian College Students." *Ethnicity and Disease* 19, no. 2): 111–4.

Phillips, R. L., L. Garfinkel, J. W. Kuzma, W. L. Beeson, T. Lotz, and B. Brin. "Mortality among California Seventh-Day Adventists for Selected Cancer Sites." *Journal of the National Cancer Institute* 65, no. 5 (1980): 1097–1107.

Phillips, R.L., F. R. Lemon, W. L. Beesonm and J. W. Kuzma. "Coronary Heart Disease Mortality among Seventh-Day Adventists with Differing Dietary Habits: A Preliminary Report." *American Journal of Clinical Nutrition* 31, no. 10 supplement (1978): S191-S198.

Powell, Lisa M., Sandy Slater, Donka Mirtcheva, Yanjun Bao, and Frank J. Chaloupka. "Food Store Availability and Neighborhood Characteristics in the United States." *Preventative Medicine* 44, no. 3 (2007): 189–95.

Pozio, E., O. Cappelli, L. Marchesi, P. Valeri, P. Rossi. "Third Outbreak of Trichinellosis Caused by Consumption of Horse Meat in Italy." *Annales de Parasitologie Humaine et Comparee* 63, no. 1 (1988): 48–53.

Prato, Rosa, Pier Luigi Lopalco, Maria Chironna, Giovanna Barbuti, Cinzia Germinario, and Michele Quarto. "Norovirus Gastroenteritis General Outbreak Associated with Raw Shellfish Consumption in South Italy." *BMC Infectious Diseases* 4 no. 37. doi: 10.1186/1471–2334–4–37

Sabaté, Joan. "Nut Consumption, Vegetarian Diets, Ischemic Heart Disease Risk, and All-cause Mortality: Evidence from Epidemiologic Studies." *American Journal of Clinical Nutrition* 70, no. 3 supplement (1999): 500S-503S.

Salti, Ibrahim, Eric Bénard, Bruno Detournay, Monique Bianchi-Biscay, Corinne Le Brigand, Céline Voinet, Abdul Jabbar. "A Population-based Study of Diabetes and Its Characteristics During the Fasting Month of Ramadan in 13 Countries: Results of the Epidemiology of Diabetes and Ramadan 1422/2001 (EPIDIAR) Study." *Diabetes Care* 27, no. 10 (2004): 2306–11.

Schellenberg, Roberta S., Ben J. K. Tan, James D. Irvine, Donna R. Stockdale, Alvin A. Gajadhar, Bouchra Serhir, Juri Botha, Cheryl A. Armstrong, Shirley A. Woods, Joseph M. Blondeau, and Tammy L. McNab. "An Outbreak of Trichinellosis Due to Consumption of Bear Meat Infected with Trichinella Nativa, in 2 Northern Saskatchewan Communities." *Journal of Infectious Diseases* 188, no. 6 (2003): 835–43.

Schultz, Myron G., John A. Hermos, and James H. Steele. "Epidemiology of Beef Tapeworm Infection in the United States." *Public Health Reports* 85, no. 2 (1970): 169–76.

Snowdon, D.A., R. L. Phillips, and G. E. Fraser. "Meat Consumption and Fatal Ischemic Heart Disease." *Preventative Medicine* 13, no. 5 (1984): 490–500.

Snowdon, David A. and Roalnd L. Phillips. "Does A Vegetarian Diet Reduce the Occurrence of Diabetes?" *American Journal of Public Health* 75, no. 5 (1985): 507–12.

Strachan, D. P., K. J. Powell, A. Thaker, F. J. Millard, and J. D. Maxwell. "Vegetarian Diet as a Risk Factor for Tuberculosis in Immigrant South London Asians." *Thorax* 50, no. 2 (1995): 175–80.

Takeuchi, Masakazu, Kousuke Okamoto, Tatsuya Takagi, Hitoshi Ishii. "Ethnic Difference in Inter-East Asian Subjects with Normal Glucose Tolerance and Impaired Glucose Regulation: A Systematic Review and Meta-analysis Focusing on Fasting Serum Insulin." *Diabetes Research and Clinical Practice* 82, no. 3 (2008): 383–90.

Temizhan, A., O. Dönderici, D. Ouz, and B. Demirbas. "Is There Any Effect of Ramadan Fasting on Acute Coronary Heart Disease Events?" *International Journal of Cardiology* 70, no. 2 (1999): 149–53.

Tonstad, Serena, Terry Butler, Ru Yan, Gary E. Fraser. "Type of Vegetarian Diet, Body Weight, and Prevalence of Type 2 Diabetes." *Diabetes Care* 32, no. 5 (2009): 791–6.

Villegas, Raquel, Xiao Ou Shu, Yu-Tang Gao, Gong Yang, Tom Elasy, Honglan Li, and Wei Zheng. "Vegetable but Not Fruit Consumption Reduces the Risk of Type 2 Diabetes in Chinese Women." *Journal of Nutrition* 138, no. 3 (2008): 574–80.

Wang, Jing, Haiyu Qi, Zongli Diao, Xiaoyan Zheng, Xiaoli Li, Suxia Ma, Aiping Ji, and Chenghong Yin. "An Outbreak of Angiostrongyliasis Cantonensis in Beijing." *Journal of Parasitology* 96, no. 2 (2010): 377–381.

Willett, Walter. "Lessons from Dietary Studies in Adventists and Questions for the Future." *American Journal of Clinical Nutrition* 78 supplement (2003): 539S-43S.

World Health Organization: Avian Influenza Food Safety Issues. "Is It Safe to Eat Chicken?" http://www.who.int/foodsafety/micro/avian/en/index1.html

World Health Organization, "Food Safety and Food Handling." http://www.who.int/foodsafety/micro/avian/en/index1.html#handling.

Wu, Anna H., Mimi C. Yu, Chiu-Chen Tseng, Frank Z. Stanczyk, and Malcom C. Pike. "Dietary Patterns and Breast Cancer Risk in Asian American Women." *American Journal of Clinical Nutrition* 89, no. 4 (2009): 1145–54.

Yipintsoi, T., A. Lim, and W. Jintapakorn. "Prevalence of Cardiovascular Risk Factors in a Rural Area in Southern Thailand: Potential Ethnic Differences." *Journal of the Medical Association of Thailand* 88, no. 2 (2005): 196–204.

Yoshikawa, Masahide, Mariko Nishiofuku, Kei Moriya, Yukiteru Ouji, Shigeaki Ishizaka, Kei Kasahara, Kei-ichi Mikasa, Toshiko Hirai, Youka Mizuno, Shuhei Ogawa, Takahito Nakamura, Haruhiko Maruyama, and Nobuaki Akao. "A Familial Case of Visceral Toxocariasis Due to Consumption of Raw Bovine Liver." *Parasitology International* 57, no. 4 (2008): 525–9.

DIETARY PRACTICES:

BUDDHIST:

Buddha Dharma Education Association, Inc. *Buddhanet*. http://www.buddhanet.net/index.html

Buddhist Dietary Customs http://www.clovegarden.com/diet/buddha.html

Epstein, Ron. "Resources for the Study of Buddism." http://online.sfsu.edu/~rone/Buddhism/Buddhism.htm

Ohlsson, Michael. *The Buddhist Diet* http://online.sfsu.edu/~rone/Buddhism/Buddhist%20Diet.htm

"The Five Contemplations When Eating" http://www.bhaisa-jyaguru.com/buddhist-ayurveda-encyclopedia/five_contemplations_when_eating_wu-gwan.htm

Weintraub, Eileen. "Life as a Vegetarian Tibetan Buddhist Practioner: A Personal View." http://www.serv-online.org/Eileen-Weintraub.htm

THE CHURCH OF JESUS CHRIST OF LATTER-DAY SAINTS

The Book of Mormon http://scriptures.lds.org/en/bm/contents

The Doctrine and Covenants http://scriptures.lds.org/en/dc/contents

The LDS Word of Wisdom Internet Page http://www.lds.org/ldsorg/v/index.jsp?index=23&locale=0&sourceId=0692f73c28d98010VgnVCM1000004d82620a&vgnextoid=bbd508f54922d010VgnVCM1000004d82620aRCRD (Be sure to read the following subsections for supplementary insights into the LDS Word of Wisdom: Additional Information,

Scripture References, Church Magazine Articles, and Additional On-line Materials.)

HINDUISM

"Ayurveda Foods." http://www.rajasthanvisit.com/ayurveda-food.htm

Bhagavad-Gita. http://www.bhagavad-gita.org/index-english. html (Be sure to read the commentaries by the four authorized Vaisnava Sampradayas for additional interpretation of scriptures.)

Jayaram, V. "Hinduism and Food." http://hinduwebsite.com/hinduism/h_food.asp

Bloomfield, Maurice, trans. *Hymns of the Atharva Veda* http://www.sacred-texts.com/hin/av.htm

Buhler, G., trans. *Manusmriti* http://www.hindubooks.org/manusmriti.pdf

Maharishi, Kaviyogi, trans. "Project Madurai: Thirukkural in Tamil." http://www.tamilnation.org/literature/Kural/kavi-yogi/tksindex.htm

"The Story of the Fortunate One." *Srimad Bhagavatam* http://www.srimadbhagavatam.org/

JUDAISM

Rich, Tracey R. "Judaism 101." http://www.jewfaq.org/index.htm

My Jewish Learning http://www.myjewishlearning.com/

Project Genesis, Inc. http://www.Torah.org

ISLAM

"Halal/Haraam" http://special.worldofislam.info/Food/halal_haram.html

Islam 101 http://www.islam101.com

"Raising Awareness of FIQH and ULAMAA." *Islamic-Laws.com* http://www.islamic-laws.com/halalharamfooddrinks.htm

University of Southern California. *The Qur'an.* Center for Muslim and Jewish Engagement http://www.usc.edu/schools/college/crcc/engagement/resources/texts/muslim/quran/

THE SEVENTH-DAY ADVENTIST CHURCH

Seventh-day Adventist Church Manual, Revised 2005, 17th Ed. http://www.adventist.org/beliefs/church_manual/index. html

Seventh-day Adventist Dietetic Association http://www.sdada.org

Seventh-day Adventist Guidelines http://www.adventist.org/ beliefs/guidelines/index.html

Seventh-day Adventist Official Statements http://www.adventist. org/beliefs/statements/index.html

Seventh-day Adventist Position statement on Vegetarians Diets http://www.sdada.org/position.htm

White, Ellen G. Collected Writings. Ellen G. White Estate, Inc. http://www.whiteestate.org/

FASTING

Bhagavad-Gita. http://www.bhagavad-gita.org/index-english. html

Blondheim, D. S., O. Blondheim, and S. H. Blondheim. "The Dietary Composition of Pre-fast Meals and Its Effect on 24 Hour Food and Water Fasting." *Israeli Medical Association Journal* 3, no. 9 (2001): 657–62.

Dhammapada http://www.thebigview.com/download/dham-mapada.pdf

Hadith http://www.usc.edu/schools/college/crcc/engagement/ resources/texts/muslim/hadith/

Holy Bible http://www.biblegateway.com/versions/King-James-Version-KJV-Bible/

Seventh-day Adventist Church Manual, Revised 2005, 17th Ed. http://www.adventist.org/beliefs/church_manual/index. html

"The Noble Eightfold Path." http://www.thebigview.com/bud-dhism/eightfoldpath.html

University of Southern California. *The Qur'an*. Center for Muslim and Jewish Engagement http://www.usc.edu/ schools/college/crcc/engagement/resources/texts/muslim/ quran/

IRRITABLE BOWEL SYNDROM

International Foundation for Functional Gastrointestinal Disorders website http://www.aboutibs.org

Medline Plus, A Service of the U.S. National Library of Science and the National Institutes of Health website http://www.nlm.nih.gov/medlineplus/irritablebowelsyndrome.html

National Digestive Disease Information Clearinghouse website http://digestive.niddk.nih.gov/ddiseases/pubs/ibs_ez/

WOW DIET RULES

Anderson, C. A. and C. L. Berseth. "Neither Motor Responses Nor Gastric Emptying Vary in Response to Formula Temperature in Preterm Infants." *Biology of the Neonate* 70, no. 5 (1996): 265–70.

Bateman, D. N. "Effects of Meal Temperature and Volume on the Emptying of Liquid from the Human Stomach." *Journal of Physiology* 331 (1982): 461–7.

Berkey, C. S., H. R. Rockett, M. W. Gillman, A. E. Field, and G. A. Colditz. "Longitudinal Study of Skipping Breakfast and Weight Change in Adolescents." *International Journal of Obesity Related Metabobolic Disorders* 27, no. 10 (2003): 1258–1266.

Centers for Disease Control. "Q&A: E. Coli Sickness." http://www.cdc.gov/ecoli/qa_ecoli_sickness.htm

Cho, Sungsoo, Marion Dietrich, Coralie J. P. Brown, Celeste A. Clark, and Gladys Block. "The Effect of Breakfast Type on Total Daily Energy Intake and Body Mass Index: Results from the Third National Health and Nutrition Examiniation Survey (NHANES III)." *Journal of the American College of Nutrition* (2003): 296–302.

Koebnick, C., I. Wagner, P. Leitzmann, U. Stern, and H. J. Zunft. "Probiotic Beverage Containing Lactobacillus Casei Shirota Improves Gastrointestinal Symptoms in Patients with Chronic Constipation." *Canadian Journal of Gastroenterology* 17, no. 11 (2003): 655–59.

Koletzko, Berthold and André Michael Toschke. "Meal Patterns and Frequencies: Do They Affect Body Weight in

Children and Adolescents?" *Critical Reviews in Food Science Nutrition* 50, no. 2 (2010): 100–5.

Lowe, M. R., R. A. Annunziato, J. T. Markowitz, E. Didie, D. L. Bellace, L. Riddell, C. Maille, S. McKinney, and E. Stice. "Multiple Types of Dieting Prospectively Predict Weight Gain During the Freshman Year of College." *Appetite* 47, no. 1 (2006): 83–90.

Ma, Y., E. R. Bertone, E. J. Stanek, G. W. Reed, J. R. Hebert, N. L. Cohen, P. A. Merriam, and I. S. Ockene. "Association Between Eating Patterns and Obesity in a Free-living US Adult Population." *American Journal of Epidemiology* 158, no. 1 (2003): 85–92.

McArthur, Katherine E. and Mark Feldman. "Gastric Acid Secretion, Gastrin Release and Gastric Emptying Following Ingestion of Hot, Warm or Cold coffee in Humans [Abstract]." *Gastroenterology* 90 (1986): 1540.

Möllenbrink, M. and E. Bruckschen. "Treatment of Chronic Constipation with Physiologic Escherichia coli Bacteria. Results of a Clinical Study of the Effectiveness and Tolerance of Microbiological Therapy with the E. coli Nissle 1917 Strain (Mutaflor)." *Medizinische Klinik* 89, no. 11 (1994): 587–93.

Neumark-Sztainer, Dianne, Melanie Wall, Jia Guo, Mary Story, Jess Haines, and Marla Eisenberg. "Obesity, Disordered Eating, and Eating Disorders in a Longitudinal Study of Adolescents: How Do Dieters Fare 5 Years Later?" *Journal of the American Dietetic Association* 106, no. 4 (2006): 559–68.

Neumark-Sztainer, Dianne, Melanie Wall, Mary Story, Jess Haines, and Marla Eisenberg. "Why Does Dieting Predict Weight Gain in Adolescents? Findings from Project EAT-II: A 5-year Longitudinal Study." *Journal of the American Dietetic Association* 107(3): 448–55.

Rideout, Candice A. and Susan I. Barr. " 'Restrained Eating' versus 'Trying to Lose Weight': How Are They Associated with Body Weight and Tendency to Overeat among Postmenopausal women?" *Journal of the American Dietetic*

Association 109, no. 5 (2009): 890–93.

Shi, X., W. Bartoli, M. Horn, R. Murray. "Gastric Emptying of Cold Beverages in Humans: Effect of Transportable Carbohydrates." *Interational Journal of Sports, Nutrition, Exercise, and Metabolism* 10, no. 4 (2000): 394–403.

Szajewska, Hania and Marek Ruszczynski. "Systemic Review Demonstrating that Breakfast Consumption Influences Body Weight Outcomes in Children and Adolescents in Europe." *Critical Reviews in Food Science Nutrition* 50, no. 2 (2010): 113–119.

Tiggemann, Marika. "Dietary Restraint and Self-esteem as Predictors of Weight Gain Over an 8-year Time Period." *Eating Behaviors* 5, no. 3 (2004): 251–9.

Toschke, A. M., K. H. Thorsteinsdottir, R. Von Kries, GME Study Group. "Meal Frequency, Breakfast Consumption and Childhood Obesity." *International Journal of Pediatric Obesity* 4, no. 4 (2009): 242–248.

USDA "Milk Tips." Food Pyramid. http://www.pyramid.gov/pyramid/milk_tips.html

Yang, Yue-Xin, Mei He, Gang Hu, Jie Wei, Philippe Pages, Xian=Hua Yang, and Sophie Bourdu-Naturel. "Effect of a Fermented Milk Containing *Bifidobacterium lactis* DN-173010 on Chinese Constipated Women." *World Journal of Gastroenterology* 14, no. 40 (2008): 6237–43.

MISCELLANEOUS

Alfenas, Rita C. G. and Richard D. Mattes. "Influence of Glycemic Index/Load on Glycemic Response, Appetite, and Food Intake in Healthy Humans." *Diabetes Care* 28, no. 9 (2005): 2123–29.

American Dental Association website http://www.ada.org/public/topics/diet.asp

American Dietetic Association website http://www.eatright.org/Public/

Aston, L. M., C. S. Stokes, S. A. Jebb. "No Effect of a Diet with a Reduced Glycaemic Index on Satiety, Energy Intake and Body Weight in Overweight and Obese Women."

International Journal of Obesity (London) 32, No. 1 (2008): 160–5.

Avena, Nicole M., Pedro Rada, and Bartley G. Hoebel. "Evidence for Sugar Addiction: Behavioral and Neurochemical Effects of Intermittent, Excessive Sugar Intake." *Neuroscience and Biobehavioral Reviews* 32 (2008): 20–29.

Avena, Nicole M., Pedro Rada, and Bartley G. Hoebel. "Sugar and Fat Bingeing Have Notable Differences in Addictive-like Behavior." *Journal of Nutrition* 139 (2009): 623–628.

Ball, Shauna D., Kelly R. Keller, Laurie J. Moyer-Mileur, Yi-Wen Ding, David Donaldson, W. Daniel Jackson. "Prolongation of Satiety after Low Versus Moderately High Glycemic Index Meals in Obese Adolescents." *Pediatrics* 111, no. 3 (2003): 488–94.

Burton-Freeman, Britt. "Dietary Fiber and Energy Regulation." *Journal of Nutrition* 130 supplement (2000): 272S–5.

Corsica, Joyce A. and Bonnie J. Spring. "Carbohydrate-craving: A Double-blind, Placebo-controlled Test of the Self-medication Hypothesis." *Eating Behaviors* 4 (2008): 447–454.

Corsica, Joyce A. and Marcia L. Pelchat. "Food Addiction: True or False?" *Current Opinion in Gastroenterology* 26 (2010): 165–169.

Cote, Susan, Paul Gletman, Martha Nunn, Kathy Lituri, Michelle Henshaw, and Raul I. Garcie. "Dental Caries of Refugee Children Compared with US Children." *Pediatrics* 114, no. 6 (2004): e733-e740. doi: 10.1542/peds.2004–0496.

Ernst, E. "Iridology: A Systematic Review." *Forsch Komplementarmed* 6, no. 1 (1999): 7–9.

Ernst. E. "Iridology: Not Useful and Potentially Harmful." *Archives of Opthalmology* 118, no. 1 (2000): 120–121.

Howarth, Nancy C., Edward Saltzman, and Susan B. Roberts. "Dietary Fiber and Weight Regulation." *Nutrition Reviews* 59 (2001): 129 –39.

Ifland, J. R., H. G. Preuss, M. T. Marcus, K. M. Rourke, W. C. Taylor, K. Burau, W. S. Jacobs, W. Kadish, and G. Manso G. "Refined Food Addiction: A Classic Substance

Use Disorder." *Medical Hypotheses* 72, no. 5 (2009): 518–26.

Isaksson, Hannah, Birgitta Sundberg, Per Aman, Helena Fredriksson, and Johan Olsson. "Whole Grain Rye Porridge Breakfast Improves Satiety Compared to Refined Wheat Bread Breakfast." *Food & Nutrition Research* (2008). doi: 10.3402/fnr.v52i0.1809.

Jiménez-Cruz, A., A. N. Gutiérrez-González, and M. Bacardi-Gascon. "Low Glycemic Index Lunch on Satiety in Overweight and Obese People with Type 2 Diabetes." *Nutricion Hospitalaria* 20, no. 5 (2005): 348–50.

Jiménez-Cruz A, V. Manuel Loustaunau-López, and M. Bacardi-Gascón. "The Use of Low Glycemic and High Satiety Index Food Dishes in Mexico: A Low Cost Approach to Prevent and Control Obesity and Diabetes." *Nutricion Hospitalaria* 21, no. 3 (2006): 353–6.

Knipschild, Paul. "Looking for Gall Bladder Disease in the Patient's Iris." *BMJ: British Medical Journal* 297, no. 6663 (1988): 1578–1581.

MacGregor, Alexander B. "Diet and Dental Disease in Ghana." *Annals of the Royal College of Surgeons of England* 34 (1964): 79–185.

Munstedt, K., S. El-Safadi, F. Bruck, M. Zygmunt, A. Hackethal, and H. R. Tinneberg. "Can Iridology Detect Susceptibility to Cancer? A Prospective Case Control Study." *Journal of Alternative and Complementary Medicine* 11, no. 3 (2005): 515–519.

Pal, Sebely, Siew Lim, and Garry Egger. "The Effect of a Low Glycaemic Index Breakfast on Blood Glucose, Insulin, Lipid Profiles, Blood Pressure, Body Weight, Body Composition and Satiety in Obese and Overweight Individuals: A Pilot Study." *Journal of the American College of Nutrition* 27, no. 3 (2008): 387–93.

Pelchat, Marcia Levin. "Food Addiction in Humans." *The Journal of Nutrition* 139 (2009): 620–622.

Putnam, J. and J. Allshouse. "U.S. Per Capita Food Supply Trends." US Department of Agriculture http://www.ers.

usda.gov/publications/foodreview/sep1998/frsept98a.pdf

Rolls, Barbara J., Julia A. Ello-Martin, and Beth Carlton Tohill. "What Can Intervention Studies Tell Us about the Relationship between Fruit and Vegetable Consumption and Weight Management?" *Nutrition Reviews* 62 (2004): 1–17.

Sgan-Cohen, H. D., D. Steinberg, S. P. Zusman, and M. N. Sela. "Dental Caries and Its Determinants among Recent Immigrants from Rural Ethiopia." *Community Dentistry and Oral Epidemiology* 20 (1992): 338–342.

Simmon, Allie, David M. Worthen, and John A. Mitas. "An Evaluation of Iridology." *JAMA* 242, no. 13 (1979): 1385–1389.

Spring, Bonnie, Kristin Schneider, Malaina Smith, Darla Kendzor, Bradley Appelhans, Donald Hedeker, and Sherry Pagoto. "Abuse Potential of Carbohydrate for Overweight Carbohydrate Cravers." *Psychopharmacology* 197, no. 4 (2008): 637–647.

U.S. Department of Agriculture. *The Food Pyramid* http://www.mypyramid.gov/

Venugopal, T., V. S. Kulkarni, R. A. Nerurker, S. G. Damie, P. N. Patnekar. "Epidemiological Study of Dental Caries." *Indian Journal of Pediatrics* 65, no. 6 (1998): 883–889.

Warren, Janet M., C. Jeya Henry, and Vanessa Simonite. "Low Glycemic Index Breakfasts and Reduced Food Intake in Preadolescent Children." *Pediatrics* 112 (2003): e414.

Weston A. Price Foundation Comments to the FDA Obesity Working Group Reference Docket Number 2003N-0338 page 22. http://www.fda.gov/OHRMS/DOCKETS/dockets/03n0338/03N-0338_emc-000043–01.pdf

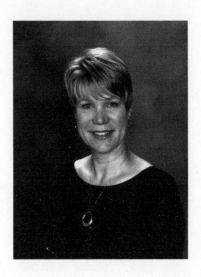

ABOUT THE AUTHOR

Michelle is a graduate of Arizona State University, Utah State University, and the University of Utah. She has published three books and over twenty-five articles in peer-reviewed professional journals. Michelle and her family happily reside in Utah.

PLEASE VISIT MICHELLE'S WEBSITE:

WWW.MICHELLE-SNOW.COM